Schizoaffective:
Evolution of My Illness

Randal Doering

This book is a work of non-fiction, but I have changed all names into fictitious names, except when I had permission to use the real names.

The cover photo comes from the web-based image exchange Dreamstime. It was done by Maksim Pasco and is titled "Fire Angel."

ISBN: 1977869270
ISBN-13: 978-1977869272

This book is dedicated to the psychiatrists and psychologists who have treated my illness over the years.

Schizoaffective disorder is a mental illness that shares the psychotic symptoms of schizophrenia and the mood disturbances of depression or bipolar disorder.

-   **The Free Dictionary/Medical Dictionary**

ACKNOWLEDGEMENTS

If you want to find the latest information on schizoaffective disorder, psychiatric medicines and their side effects, psychotic symptoms, resources for the mentally ill, just use any internet search engine. In a few instances, where the information on the web is durable, I listed some web sites below.

As always when writing a book, I consulted dictionary.com and thesaurus.com to more precisely define words for which I had a general meaning and wanted something more specific.

Here are the major sources I used to research this memoir:

Psychcentral.com schizoaffective forums	web site; very useful
"Living with Schizoaffective Disorder"	Michael Crawford on Psychcentral.com
Beating the Adversary	Richard David Price
Darkness Visible	William Styron
Icarus Redeemed: A Schizoaffective Story	G. H. Francis
Randal, Randal, Burning Bright	Randal Doering
Saving Normal	Allen Frances
Schizoaffective Disorder: Victory is Possible	Lacy Wise
The Center Cannot Hold: My Journey Through Madness	Elyn Saks
What a Life Can Be: One Therapist's Take On Schizo-Affective Disorder	Carolyn Dobbins, PhD

CONTENTS

Foreword   xi

Prologue   xiii

September: nine long years   16

October: don't you want a girlfriend?   34

November: delusions   61

December: merry fucking Christmas   76

January 2016: crawling out of the slime   87

February: someday things will be better   96

March: a cure is near?   103

April: hypomanic showers…   114

May: …bring story ideas   123

June: dad's birthday   132

July: Heather   142

August: brain tumor   152

September: thoughts from friends   164

October: what scares you   175

November: light the fuse and run   182

December: nothing but a murderer   199

January 2017: asymmetric warfare   211

February: the victor   227

Epilogue   240

About the Author   241

Foreword

This is a book about mental illness. It is not a medical book, full of psychiatric musings; nor is it a case history, in dry medical language. This book is a memoir, filled with the experiences and the horrors of my illness. My purpose in writing it is to show how my schizoaffective disorder evolved over 18 months. Some delusions persisted over time, and others changed every few months. Hallucinations came and went but were almost always unpleasant, and sometimes they occurred so often and so loud that they filled my mind for days or even months on end. Manic spikes, accompanied by insomnia and spending sprees, reduced me to near-idiocy, and the voices in my head hounded and belittled me for a year and a half.

The story has heroes. There are shrinks in the background of the tale, tweaking dosages and trying new medications as old ones became ineffective. Friends and family members supported me by asking as to my health, and friends who were mentally ill suggested ways to fight the symptoms.

Most mental illness memoirs follow an arc: the narrator becomes mentally ill and suffers some embarrassments due to their symptoms. There is a hint of the possibility of suicide, just to raise the stakes. The narrator finds their way into therapy, and after a while they become well and return to their interrupted life.

In this memoir I offer no such arc to recovery. There is a sizeable percentage of mentally ill people who do not get better. Their illness is chronic, and the symptoms continue despite medication changes and therapeutic interventions. I wrote this book to give you, the reader, a realistic view of how schizoaffective disorder changes and adapts as a long-term condition. It is not meant to be bleak but to be real. I hope it is of value to you.

Prologue

Mental illness comes, mental illness goes. In my first memoir, *Randal, Randal, Burning Bright*, I laid out the course of my journey from vague mental difficulties to full-blown psychological disorder. The book covered four years and followed my path through illness, job loss, homelessness, attempted suicide, and finally psychiatric intervention and something like recovery. At the end of the book it looked like I had defeated the illness, and I headed back to California to spend time with friends and try to start over again.

Things didn't work out. Within a few months of returning to San Francisco the psychotic episodes began again, and my head filled with voices and paranoia once more. As a psychotic, I couldn't find work. My friends felt uncomfortable at the weird things I said when I was psychotic, and they abandoned me. My disability payments started, so I didn't become homeless again, and I turned to the VA clinic in San Francisco for psychiatric help. The VA assigned me a psychiatrist, and we worked with the medicines and the dosages and tried to find a cure. As time went on it became clear that the illness followed a cycle. There would be six or eight months of bad symptoms, vicious and beyond control of the medication, and then there would be a couple months when the illness would lighten up, and I would become hopeful that it would go completely away.

Then the bad months would return again. This went on for years, and nothing I tried made the situation any better. There would be no miracle cure, no dramatic intervention that would save me, no end to the voices and the hallucinations and all the rest of the ugly symptoms that defined my world.

I lived in San Francisco for over a year, but that city is terribly costly, and I was forced out by the high prices. I moved to San Diego, which is cheaper. I discovered that there are these places,

Single Room Occupancy (SRO) hotels, where rent is cheap and cockroaches are common. The idea is, you rent a single room, and you buy a mini-fridge and a microwave oven so you can eat in your room. I started doing a little creative writing, an hour a day, and finished a novel that I had been working on for over a decade. I shopped it around, but no agents or editors showed interest. After I moved to San Diego I found new friends and fought schizoaffective disorder every day in my battle to live a meaningful life.

Unfortunately, the illness didn't let up. This book, my second memoir, picks up in late 2015, seven years after the end of my first memoir.

Down Cycle

September: nine long years

"Hey, asshole. Why don't you fuck me and give me three kids?"

The young woman's voice, whispered right into my left ear, shocked me into letting go of the book I was reading. This was at a café in my neighborhood. The book fell onto a small table and snapped shut. Five o'clock in the morning, and these utterances gave me a stinging headache.

What do you want, Heather? I thought.

"I want you to move to Los Angeles and help me with my career. You're not doing anything useful. You're so fucked up most of the time you can barely find your own ass with both hands. All I need from you is your dick, and maybe you can type some press releases for me. Something valuable. You're no good to yourself, but maybe you can serve me. Think about it. Think *fast*, because if you say *no*, I'm going to punish you like the devil himself."

She became visible out of the side of my eye. Here was a twenty-something year old white woman, petite and very pretty, with long red hair and brilliant green eyes. She wore a colorful dress in shades of yellow, rust, brown, black, and bright blue, and the patches of color accentuated her breasts. The dress was artfully done; *Heather* was artfully done, and sexual thoughts percolated through my head.

"Come to L.A.," she repeated, and then, just like that, I couldn't see her anymore. I glanced around, but she wasn't there.

"I need you to make calls to editors, and find me more work," her voice stabbed in my mind. This *hurt*, and it set off a nasty headache. In moments, my world imploded into a ball of seething pain. "I *need you* to get me pregnant. You have to get a real job, none of this SSDI/disability bullshit. Support me. You need to stop reading stupid fantasy novels and start studying humorous stories in the media. Look at online humor magazines, and funny newspaper columns. PAY ATTENTION!"

I'll get my shrink to up the dosage of meds, I threatened her. *I'll make you disappear.*

"Your drugs are placebos," she jabbed. "The whole world is different from what you believe. Hollywood executives are working with your psychiatrist to dope you up on hallucinogens and keep you from realizing the truth. You stupid son of a bitch. There are more people out to get you than you ever dreamed. I'm going to show you how deep it all goes."

Then she fell silent.

This was mid-September. My illness had been quiet for months. But now Heather was rowdy, and the games were about to begin.

Once upon a time, there was a voice in my head that I named Sheila, in my first memoir. That was *Randal, Randal, Burning Bright.* In that book I called her Sheila on whim; since then she has insisted that her real name is Heather, and so I call her that for purposes of this book. Over the years Heather became *loud.* She would insert herself into my thoughts, sometimes screaming and making demands, and sometimes as a visual hallucination that seemed to have her own independent life. When she visited, bad things were on the way.

Disturbed by her promise to show me "how deep it goes," I picked up my book and my cup of coffee and took my morning walk, a mile and a half through my neighborhood. I had had several psychiatrists through the VA over the years, and all of them had urged me to take up some form of exercise as a way of pumping helpful chemicals through my brain and staying fit. Also, exercise helped me fight the voices and the delusions and the paranoia, and maybe sometimes it helped control the manic outbursts that happened so frequently.

The sun had not yet risen, and as I walked down the sidewalk, a homeless man played a small radio so quietly I could barely hear it. He sat on a low wall enclosing a flower bed, at an old age home. I couldn't hear the song from the radio, but what occurred to me instead was that the music was saying,

"Your girlfriend is risen; your Savior's on track. They're all lying to you, and holding you back."

I stared at the homeless man, and he gave me a freaked-out look. What look was on my own face? I must have looked insane. So I quickly passed him by and went on my way.

Cars cruised past, not many, all going slower than usual. No one was in a hurry, at this pre-dawn time of day.

I looked up at the skyscrapers on San Diego's skyline and saw jet planes crash into the upper floors of the buildings. There were huge explosions, and the buildings fell. A terrible sense of foreboding filled my guts. I couldn't tell if it was day or night anymore, but it was clear that I had just relived the 9/11 attacks, and in my mind thousands of people died.

Dazed, I walked through the streets of San Diego, barely able to keep to my route. Was it all going to happen again? Were there going to be more attacks, all over America? Was I remembering the past, or seeing the future?

A black sedan went past, slowly, and the vehicle passed me a message: *It's all a lie. They're experimenting on you. Drugs you've never even heard of. They've replaced your whole life with fiction. It's the New York publishing scene, and those fuckers are ruthless. Beware!*

I went home and ate some cereal and killed a few hours skimming news articles on the internet. I say 'skimming,' because that is the nature of my ability to read, these days: read and re-read, jump around on the page, go over the same material half a dozen times, and patch together some idea what the words meant.

I half expected to see more planes crash into skyscrapers, but this didn't happen. This sort of hallucination was frequent, for me. The visions occurred, I was upset for a while, and when the delusions or hallucinations didn't repeat, or no one talked about it, I let the incident go.

On Friday afternoons I volunteered at the public library for a few hours. The duties were simple: greet patrons who entered the art gallery, and keep an eye on things to make sure no one trashed the place. Some of the patrons wanted to talk about the exhibits, and others wanted to chat about past exhibits or what was coming up next, and so my volunteer hours were also a chance to socialize.

I walked to the library and sat at the desk, ready for a good experience, but I guess Heather just couldn't stand any sign that I might be enjoying myself, because she hollered and screeched:

"The New York publishers own this library! Volunteering here is throwing yourself into their trap! You want to read books? Read these words: I ALWAYS WIN IN THE END!" She made noises and sang various pop music songs as I tried to read, during the slower periods on the volunteer shift. This happened again and again, and I gritted my teeth and tried to concentrate. The shift passed, and I walked back to my room.

A few days passed. I dreamed of voices, just below my threshold of hearing. Businessmen jumped off burning skyscrapers and plummeted to their death. Heather danced in the wreckage, barely visible as a little figure far away. She was there when I went to the café, and she was there when I took my morning walk. She smiled sometimes, but it was more like a threat than a smile.

Then one morning I sat in the café. Half a dozen patrons had bought drinks and a snack; they sat far apart from each other, and no one carried on a conversation.

"There was no 9/11," said one guy, a young black man in a black hoodie. I was trying to read a book, but his voice cut into my thoughts so sharply that I closed the book and looked over at him. He was in mid-drink, literally with a cup of coffee pressed to his lips. That made me shiver. This guy hadn't said anything. I had the feeling that something was wrong, but I didn't understand what. My thoughts started to spin, and I got a headache. In the back of my mind, planes smashed into buildings, and tons of debris rained down onto the streets.

A middle-aged white guy in a black leather jacket took a bite of a bagel. In mid-chomp, he said: "Everything you've been told is a lie. Who would benefit from destroying the World Trade Center? Think about it. Not the insurance companies. Liars! Where did the money go? Who got the money?"

I don't know, I thought. *My head hurts.*

"That's because you're stupid," said an old white woman. I recognized her as one of the regular patrons. She sat at the counter by the big window, looking out on the street. I heard her talking, but her mouth was firmly closed.

Clearly these people could read my mind. They were inserting thoughts. They weren't talking, but I could hear them anyway. My headache grew more intense, and I turned back to my book and skimmed a few pages. Took a sip of coffee.

"Tell you what I'm going to do," said Heather, in my head. "I'm going to have three kids, and we'll *call* them yours. In secret I'll be fucking some Asian guy for one kid, and some black guy for another kid, and maybe I'll let you pick some Nobel prize winner sperm donor for the last kid. But you can raise them all. You'll do that for me, won't you?"

I heard the whine of jet engines, and hundreds of people screamed. I couldn't see the screaming people, but they were all around me. The plane slammed into the tower and exploded in a giant orange fireball. Bodies fell from the sky. On the street below people looked up and then ran.

"They're all lying to you," said the young black man. "It didn't go down that way. The truth is a whole lot weirder than that. You've heard of the Koch brothers? Rich old Republicans? Seen their pictures in the media?"

"Yeah," I said out loud. Sometimes it went like that, when I was caught up in the voices. Sometimes I started answering them out loud. Good way to get locked up in the looney bin, but that's the way it went, sometimes. "I know who they are," I continued.

The young black man went on: "No such guys as the Koch brothers. The media made them up. The *real* rich old conservatives aren't stupid enough to get their pictures on the news. They *own* the news. They decide what gets reported. You follow me?"

"No," I mumbled. I was looking straight at the young black guy. His mouth wasn't moving, but I heard his voice in my mind, very clearly. Who did he work for, the government? The media?

"You ever hear people talk about 9/11?" he pressed.

"Not lately," I said.

"Not in years. There was no 9/11. It was made up to fool *you*."

"The news media said we retaliated with wars in Iraq and Afghanistan," I protested. I barely mumbled, and no one looked at me. At this time of day, half the people in the café were homeless crazies. No one took a second glance at a disheveled middle-age white guy talking to himself.

"There were no wars overseas," he said. "There is only one war, and that is the war for who gets the money. America's entertainment industry elites faked 9/11. The whole thing was financed by Hollywood, and supported by false news from the Pentagon. You've heard the wars overseas cost trillions? Guess who got that cash?"

"The Koch brothers?" I asked stubbornly.

"There *are* no Koch brothers. They're just stand-ins for the real powers that be. *Hollywood* got that money. *Conservatives* got that money. Whole lot of newly-minted fat cats, coast to coast. *New York publishing executives* got that money. *You* didn't get shit. *You* were taken for a ride."

"9/11 happened *before* I went crazy," I tried to point out, but he wagged one finger at me and tut-tutted.

"The roots of your lunacy go back farther than you think," he said. "But maybe I've said too much. You don't believe me. You need to hear the *full* story." Then he stood up and left the café, and I sat there for a long time, wondering if I should take him literally, or just as a sign of my illness.

Days went by. I dreamed of the 9/11 reflecting pool monument in New York City. I had visited this and seen it first-hand. The World Trade Center was not there anymore. This was not a delusion; this was observable fact. So what should I believe, the young black man who could be working for anyone, or my own sense of reality?

Then the attacks began in earnest. I *knew* that the social security administration was going to cut off my SSDI, and fear gripped me. I would become homeless and maybe die on the streets. Hundreds of homeless people died each year in San Diego; those were the ones officials knew about. Doubtless there were many more, murdered and buried, dumped in rivers, dead in some culvert somewhere, tossed into dumpsters.

Heather bowed out, and swarms of minor voices came in.

"you owe the VA money" "your parents hate you" "you haven't written any books; you stole all your ideas from Stephen King" "you owe the IRS a million dollars" "your masters degree is a fake" "you're a loony" "there was no 9/11"

They attacked in my sleep, and they swarmed me in the café and hounded me throughout the day. These voices intensified whenever other people were around, stinging and stabbing and throwing out their one-liners. I became convinced I was going to lose my SSDI, and that the IRS was after me. I was sure my family hated me, and I was afraid to call them. All my credentials, everything I had ever achieved in life, was fake, and only psychosis was real. The voices would destroy me, but they would have a good time doing it, and I was along for the ride.

The attacks went on for ten hours a day, each voice contributing its stings, then changing the order of things and attacking again. The planes crashed into the towers, and people died. Fireballs erupted high over the streets of New York City. Or San Diego. Or both.

Voices repeated: "there are no Koch brothers" *"you* are responsible for 9/11" "the War on Terror is a fraud" "conservatives stole the money that was supposed to go for fighting terrorists" *"you* drove the planes into the towers"

These voices awakened ferocious paranoia. The cops were coming to arrest me for masterminding 9/11. Heather was in my bank accounts and funneled my money to radical feminists. Hollywood executives were making movies that were disguised versions of my first memoir; no one had paid me for the rights to use my story. The apartment manager in my building was collecting information on what packages I got in the mail, and who they were from: it wasn't clear who he was reporting to. Organized crime?

I became fearful and did not leave my room unless it was to follow my normal daily routine. I stopped taking shopping trips to the Salvation Army thrift store, or the local Goodwill thrift store, because I was afraid that the clerks at these stores were studying my buying habits and were reporting back to Heather, who would use this information to mess with my head.

My room overlooked a busy street in San Diego, and emergency vehicles frequently rushed along with horns blasting. Every time a cop car streaked by with lights flashing, I thought they were coming for me; every fire department search and rescue truck was responding to my latest psychotic outbreak; every ambulance was there to drain my blood and take samples of my flesh to benefit biotech industry executives.

Everything that happened became a source of terror. The food I bought from the grocery store was poisoned by the store employees, who were paid by the military to get rid of me before I became the most powerful mind on the planet. Vehicles went by on the street and honked, and I knew they were calling me out so overhead Predator drones could shoot missiles at me.

Back in the real world, my father had cancer; this had started out as melanoma and had spread through his body. He was undergoing chemotherapy and complained of feeling run down and weak. The chemo left him feeling sick all the time, and he was not able to do much on a daily basis.

"It's *your* fault your father has cancer," Heather insisted. "He's a conservative, and you're a liberal, and you've hated him your whole life. You have constant hateful thoughts, and that's making his cancer worse. He doesn't need chemo; he needs a loving son. You're such a worthless piece of shit!" This made me feel horrible, and I didn't know what to do except call my parents and urge my father to keep up the chemo, and fight.

The voices rallied and brought on paranoia, and Heather tortured me with guilt, and these emotions became so intense that I nearly had a breakdown. In that moment of shattered symptoms and terrified psyche, the voices changed their tune. The change was abrupt and as all-encompassing as finding out you're an orphan whose parents adopted you when you were six.

"It's all Hollywood," Heather said gleefully as I cowered in my room. "They're making a story out of your life. Let's start off with the BIG LIE. What year do you think it is? How old do you think you are?"

"I'm fifty-one," I whispered, not wanting to give anything away to the neighbors I was sure were listening on the other side of my door.

"And the year?"

"2015."

"How long have you been schizoaffective?"

"Nine long years."

She gave a cruel smile. "You think *I'm* head-fucking you... Those media people have you so jerked around you don't know WHAT is going on. It's 2005. You're 41 years old. You're young enough to get a good job, start a family, get a life. Hollywood is using you, but they're on your side. Truth! New York City publishers have been publishing your books for years. They've had the stories translated into 70 languages, and they're pushing your stories globally. And Hollywood has been buying the rights for millions of dollars, and making movies out of your stories, and your life. So far you've made over $100 million."

"Then why do I live in a single room occupancy hotel and eat frozen dinners out of a microwave?"

"Because you're not ready to receive your due yet. You have to run the race before you win the prizes! Listen to you, 'oh, I'm suffering. My disorder is so terrible.' Terrible? Try 'lucrative.' How many people do you know get paid a hundred million bucks to have a few psychotic episodes? You're not a victim, you're on the way to *glory*. Stop whining, and embrace your fantastic future!"

Later she said, "You have no free will. I design your free will. I want three kids, and you're coming to Los Angeles to help me further my career. Right now you're just a loser, but I have big plans for you. I carry all the keys to all the locks on all the vaults that hold your future. You'll do what I want. God help you if you fight me. May the Lord have mercy on your very soul."

Then she introduced me to a new game, which she called 'Buzzword Bingo.' Voices started sounding off in my mind.

Voice 1: "Contact." This was an attack, not a comment. It was said viciously, and it cut through all my other thoughts. 'Contact' meant the voices were establishing control.

Voice 2: "Khamsa." Here is the Arabic word for 'five.' In the Enneagram system of personality types, type five is the thinker. My type is four with a touch of five. The voice was letting me know they were going after my ability to think rationally. Immediately I got a headache and felt spin-headed.

Voice 3: "Everything." The voices were going to stuff my head full of memories of everything I ever screwed up, every time I ever stumbled, every time I had failed. I thought of the time when I was four or five years old and took my shirt off during the summer and got a savage sunburn, and the shame of this bad decision made my face turn red, even now.

Voice 4: "Program." Heather and these other voices were not acting randomly but were following a ten-year plan to keep me on track through all these bad years, until I received a reward.

Voice 5: "Heather." My imaginary girlfriend and dominant voice among many in my head. Heather could do as she wished; as far as I could tell she had no limitations. She owned the cops, the government, my friends, my family, and the other voices. She had 24/7 access to everything in my head, and she could share my thoughts with whoever she pleased. Heather had total control.

The voices said these catch phrases over and over, changing the order and adding dozens of other catch phrases. Thoughts and images cascaded through my mind, but they returned to Heather and her demand for three children and to come to Los Angeles.

I want to say "we" played buzzword bingo every few days, but in truth Heather played it, and the other voices played it, and my mind was the canvas they painted their program on. It wasn't that I didn't try to fight… As soon as I heard a buzzword, I began thinking, *fuck off.* Sometimes this slowed the attacks; on rare occasion the flow of buzzwords faltered or even completely stopped. But typically Heather was in the background, orchestrating the attacks. She started off softly at first, "contact" whispered just at the threshold of hearing and then other buzzwords said in louder and louder voices until I could hear nothing but cries of "program," or "mumkin," which means 'maybe' in Arabic. In buzzword bingo, 'mumkin' meant 'maybe you should marry Heather and have some kids.'

I did know, though, when I was under full-bore assault. Voices insisted there was no 9/11, and from day to day I could not tell if my memories of visiting the reflecting pools in New York City were real or false. Trillions of dollars supposedly spent on the War on Terror, gone. I was a major writer, across the planet. Media giants supposedly stole my stories, or paid me royalties I never received.

Voices whispered buzzwords in endless strings, causing me no end of misery. And through it all, I feared the cops were out to get me, the apartment manager was out to get me, my parents were telling lies about me, God Himself was out to get my father, via cancer.

I tried to act normal but could not manage it. I stopped talking to people in the café and spent as little time there as I could, just gulped down a coffee and read a little and then back to my room, where I felt safe. I talked with my friends about the conspiracies and voices that teemed in my mind, and my fiends said I should talk to my psychiatrist about these thoughts.

After comments from several friends, I rallied and visited my psychiatrist. This was at the VA hospital where I received care. Long ago I was a soldier, and veterans receive free health care for their entire lives, through the VA hospital system. I hadn't been in the Army for decades, but I was still covered.

My shrink listened to me whine and bumped up my daily dose of an anti-psychotic called Seroquel, and I went back into the fight.

Sometimes just believing you will get well will help you recover, but this was not the case with me. The increase in Seroquel seemed to help for a few days, for a week, then the symptoms returned. Planes smashed into skyscrapers. Water flowed across reflecting pools. Endless amounts of money were earmarked for a war that never happened. Buzzwords popped in my mind like popcorn, each one causing all sorts of lies and false associations.

I had a hard time thinking. Voices and paranoia and delusions began in mid-morning and continued all the rest of the day. In addition to all these many symptoms, I began having flashbacks to events I noted in my first memoir, especially living at the Life Link, in Santa Fe, New Mexico. I had experienced similar attacks there, and these had gone on for several months and then faded slowly away. Would this time repeat the same pattern, all over again? How long was this going to go on? Two months? Six? I had no way of telling.

Several times during the remaining days of September, I had a strong urge to run away from San Diego before Heather caught me and took over my mind. I fought against all these weird thoughts, and I took my medicines, and I practiced some mental techniques that psychologists from the VA had taught me. Every few days I went to the Greyhound Bus website and looked up tickets to Santa Fe, New Mexico. I had to get away from Heather. I had to escape San Diego. The voices might not be able to follow me to New Mexico. The people at the Life Link had helped me before; could they help me again? But each time I started to buy tickets, I hesitated. Tickets cost money, and I didn't have much money. I was owed millions, but I hardly had two pennies to rub together.

So I dithered, and time passed.

Paranoid delusions flooded my mind: the cops were going to frame me for drug possession, and they would work with their buddy the judge to put me away for 20 years.

Planes rammed the towers and exploded, and body parts tumbled through the sky onto the onlookers on the streets below.

The voices in my head called out numbers, beginning at a thousand and counting down, or starting at a hundred. The voices bounced around: "1000, 900, 800, 999, 600, 50, 998…" Something big was going to happen when they reached zero, and as a few days went by I knew what it was: time for violence.

I had flashbacks to a street full of cars, and the voices in my head pushed me to do maximum harm. I stood at the side of the street, with a gun in one hand, and I was going to kill a lot of people.

Were these real memories, or were they delusions? I was certain I'd remember if I shot someone, but some days I was barely sure of my own name. Someone got shot. In fact, a lot of people got shot. Or not. Which was true?

The certainty that I had shot someone became stronger, and I went back and re-read my first memoir, looking for clues. There were incidents that never made it into that book, because some of the things I had done or almost done during those three years were so fearful that I didn't include them in the book. Those events left too intense an emotional mark on me, and I couldn't share them.

One of these deleted scenes had to do with gun violence and mental illness, but I couldn't recall the details. I knew something violent had happened or almost happened, and the voices were threatening to bring it up again. What goes around comes around: once you get on a violent path, it's hard to get off again.

As the voices counted down their numbers and flashed me hints of murder, the fears that rode me day and night grew worse. My life became a mess. I dashed to the café, dashed through my morning walk, did a little writing each day. After some temporary relief from the Seroquel increase, my illness almost completely took me over, and I sent miserable emails to friends describing my symptoms. They sent back notes suggesting I give the Seroquel time to take effect, and I had to be content with that.

Near the end of the month I sat in front of my computer, in my room, and wondered: Who were the Koch brothers? Media puppets? Had they orchestrated 9/11?

"*You* orchestrated 9/11," said Heather, in a jolly tone. She was dressed in faded blue jeans with torn-out knees, and a maroon blouse which looked too big on her. "9/11 was all about *you*," she insisted.

"That doesn't even make sense," I mumbled.

"Your buddies in big media made up 9/11 to keep you in the dark as to the real story of America," she whispered. She bent down and put her hands on her knees; her blouse fell open, and I saw her tits. Nice. Tasty.

"I want some," I commented.

"Come to L.A.," she said, and straightened back up. "You can have all you like." Her long auburn hair bounced into perfect place. She was so pretty—pretty poison. "You fucking loser," she snarled, her mood changing in an instant. "I tell you, come to L.A., and you don't bite on it. You're thinking of New Mexico, but not L.A., which

is just a couple hours up the road. You want out? Not bad enough.
Buses go by, just a block from your place, every fifteen minutes. Step
in front of one. You'll get *out*."

As you've figured out by now, I have a routine I follow most
days. When you're severely mentally ill and have a hard time dealing
with reality, and even routine functioning is difficult, you establish
some anchors in your life. Some of these I have already mentioned,
like going to the café to read a book in the morning, or taking a daily
walk. Another anchor was writing a little each day. This was my only
real sense of accomplishment in my life. Most people have a job they
go to, where they perform tasks and are able to point out progress
they have made over the years, but I no longer had that milepost.
And I had no children to raise, or a steady relationship to measure.
My writing was it, and I had been working on a novel for all of 2015.

The book was entitled *Political Mommies*, and it was about Isabella
Sierra, a young Hispanic mother of two children who angers an
undead warlock, which then goes after her and her family. The book
takes place over the course of a year and is a fantasy. By the end of
September I had a rough draft of the whole novel and was letting the
book sit for September; the idea was, I'd come back to it in October
and edit the manuscript.

You might be surprised to hear that I could work coherently on a
book at all, with the incredible amount of noise going on in my head.
But like anything you do, if you do it often enough you get good at it.
I had been writing stories as a serious hobby for nearly 30 years. I
was not particularly ambitious; each day I wrote 1,000 words or
edited 5,000 words. This was in the morning, when my mental illness
symptoms were quieter and not so ferocious. This process took
about an hour each morning. The secret of my process was not
brute force or will power but simply working within the rhythms of
my illness and within the methods I had long established from
decades of self-discipline.

Here is where the voices in my head collided with my lived experience. Heather insisted that the New York City publishers had already brought out my books, but in reality I could find no evidence of this. Instead, I sent out emails to the New York publishers, trying to entice them to pick up my books and bring them to market, but I was not having any success at making this happen. I am a writer, not a salesman, and if you were going to convince some jaded literary agent to represent your book, you either needed to slip her some money, kiss her ass, or make some powerful friends to impress her. Agents will *tell* you that it's all about the quality of your writing, but this is only half the real story: Each literary agent receive many hundreds of manuscripts each year, and many of these are pretty good. Yet, the agent can only accept three or four for representation. So what does she do? She picks out the manuscripts that she feels tell the best story, and to all other authors who submitted she sends out a little form letter saying try again, your story wasn't quite what she was looking for.... And the cycle begins anew.

I had been at this for decades. I had received many form letters from agents, and half a dozen personalized comments over the years. I was a good writer, but I was not a good salesman. I could not figure out what I needed to say to get an agent to represent my work.

Instead, I focused on the creative side of the industry. I wrote stories about American Indians, who are underrepresented in speculative fiction. I wrote stories about Hispanic characters. I wrote an epic poem about a black captain of Special Forces soldiers. One of my novels had to do with a mentally ill homeless man who takes on a supernatural murderer. I wrote a collection of short stories. I put together an illustrated novel. Hell, I tried everything over three decades of writing stories. The agents didn't want any of it. So I self-published my books, and occasionally I sold a few copies, so every year I made about a hundred dollars off my writing. Just a hobby.

The countdown voices grew loud and screeching. What had seemed like a countdown to violence morphed into a countdown to involuntary confinement. I was going to end up at the laughing academy, in a straight-jacket, so doped up I would have to be fed with a tube. I had been admitted to a mental institution before, in Egypt in 2007. This wasn't a bad experience, but that had been 'voluntary' committal. I didn't want to end up in an American mental hospital, with Nurse Ratched in command.

I began grasping for straws. How long were these symptoms going to go on? I had been through similar attacks before, years ago, and they went on for half a year. I didn't want to suffer these horrors for six months. I wasn't going to last that long. Every day was a miserable series of battles that I usually lost. Heather danced through my mind, screaming, "Come to L.A. Bring some sperm! I want babies!" She shook her butt and shivered her tits and stamped her feet, and I was perpetually on the verge of screaming, in an attempt to drive her off.

My appearance changed. I couldn't remember how long I had been wearing the same clothes, and days passed between showers. A friend complained that I "smelled funny." I changed clothes once in ten days. I wasn't sure how often I attended to hygiene. The voices became my world.

Planes slammed into towers. Fireballs. Debris. The smiling faces of the Koch brothers seemed to speak directly to me, and they said, "We own you."

It seemed important to get the facts about 9/11, and so I went online. I sort of ingested the news stories, and one of them made my brain darken with dismay. Everyone knows that the two big towers fell on that fatal day, but there was an article that said a smaller building on the periphery of the twin towers also fell. The symbolism was so obvious that even I, with my messed up head, could see it: a daddy tower, a mama tower, and a baby tower.

9/11 was Heather trying to get my attention, all those years ago!

I had a spiritual moment: the terrorists were agents of fate, and they carried out not an Islamic agenda, but an agenda of Heather.

I typed my own name into Google, and all sorts of stuff came up, but nothing about 9/11 and Heather or the Koch brothers or me with a large sum of money.

"You never wrote any books," said a voice in my head. "You found free books on Smashwords, downloaded them, and put your name on them. Fraud. Wait until the lawyers find out."

There were violent paranoid delusions: a dozen cops in riot gear ran up the stairs of my building and kicked in my door and beat the hell out of me, then dragged me off to prison. Sometimes this was due to my having stolen other people's books, and sometimes it was because I believed in 9/11 in spite of the voices insisting that it had never happened. Or maybe it had happened, but not the way I thought it had. Sometimes in these delusions I had a gun, or a submachine gun, and I died in a shootout with the cops. The context of these delusions was so blurry that I could never really tell what was going on. Did someone want to kill me? Or was it the funny farm next? Who made that determination? Heather? The cops? Me?

I took to muttering *fuck off* a dozen times a day, trying to fight Heather or the other voices, struggling to resist the Koch brothers. Sometimes I raised my voice, growling, *"Fuck off!"* as I walked down the sidewalk, and sometimes it was just me, screaming in my own mind as the voices carried on their latest countdown.

At the end of September I got on the computer and found a list of the richest people in America. I figured if I was really worth $100 million, I should be on the list. It took a while to scan the article, because my brain was not working well enough to perform a search, but the conclusion was clear: I was not there. I was worth nothing.

October: don't you want a girlfriend?

I looked forward to Halloween, because I live near the Gaslamp area of San Diego, which is the entertainment district, and every year all sorts of people dress up in wild costumes on the holiday and parade around downtown, showing off. This is fun to watch, and I wanted to see it. So I tried to ignore the voices and the countdowns and Heather and the hallucinatory cops and the homeless people out to get me, and concentrate on the positive aspects of my life.

In this endeavor I was unsuccessful. Oh, the gratitude I felt for writing 1,000 words a day was real enough, and I was pleased that I could go to Free Tuesday at the San Diego Museum of Art, and of course I was glad for the hiking trips I took with friends. I was grateful for having some good friends who put up with my complaints about my illness.

But you see, the illness didn't rest. I *knew* that those same friends were colluding with my parents and my brother to keep me sick. They had lengthy phone conversations about me, they traded emails and sent letters and postcards about me. It wasn't enough that I suffered all these symptoms; they wanted me to become so sick that I would lose touch with reality completely and became a slobbering idiot stuffed full of meds and strapped down to a chair in some nut house, drooling and giggling and gibbering.

You're asking, why would they do this? What kind of friends and family would bring such a terrible fate upon anyone? You already know the answer; I already told you. It's the money. One hundred million dollars. And of course, my family would take over my finances and "manage" them for me. Sure. My parents would buy out my friends and learn from them what *really* freaks me out, and use that to keep me down for the rest of my life. I would never escape that nut house, never get out of the straight jacket, never return to normal. And my parents would spend that money on a mansion, and servants, and fancy cars. There might even be enough money for all the aunts and uncles, all the cousins; everyone. It was going to be the biggest party in family history, and I would finance it from the living death of total mental illness implosion.

"Fuck!" Heather shrieked. "Your parents are bastards! That's *our* money, fuck bag! You can't let them get away with this!" But she was grinning, and just behind her, faded and indistinct, I could see my parents dressed up in their Sunday finest. Heather was in it with them. She was already staking a claim on my cash.

"How many kids do I want?" she belted out.

"I don't care," I growled. Was this at the café? Or on my daily walk? Or in my room? One place bled into another, and only mental illness was real.

"Run!" Heather burst out. I couldn't see her, only hear her. It was like she lived in the back of my head, and now she tried to push my brain out my forehead. "Run to Los Angeles! Look for me there! I'll guide you, you lazy piece of shit. I want kids! GIVE ME THREE KIDS!"

She punched through my mental defenses, and I ran around my room, banging off the furniture, desperate to escape the daily demands for kids. "God *damn* it, I'm too old for having kids," I yelped. "That ship done sailed!"

"Never too old, if you have the right partner. And you're not 51, you're only 41; I told you that already. Get used to it! Plenty of time left for you. GET YOUR SHIT TOGETHER! Run! Run! Run!"

I got on the computer and went to the Greyhound bus site and checked out tickets to Santa Fe, New Mexico. As the information came back, I planned out what to take. While I was doing all this, Heather howled, "Run! Run! Before the cops get you!"

The cops were on the stairs, pounding up to my room. I could *hear* them, I could *sense* their life energy, I could *feel* the vibrations of their boots slamming down on the floor. It didn't matter what I had done; it didn't matter that I hadn't *done* anything. The cops worked for Heather, and she'd use them against me as she wanted.

I sat there for several long minutes, Heather screaming in my ear, as the cops moved into position. My whole body began to shake with fear. Then I closed the internet browser on my computer and waited. My heart pounded. I heard someone tap on my door.

"Who is it?" I called out.

"Police. Open up."

Very slowly, so slowly it was hard to say I moved at all, I got up from the desk and went and opened the door.

No one was there.

I stuck my head out into the hall and glanced around. No one.

"Marry me," Heather said gently. "Or else."

"Fuck off," I hissed, and she left for a while.

The first week of October rolled on. At some point I rode a city bus, going where I do not remember, and there were ten or twelve people on board who were all talking about me:

"Going to the market," said one old Asian woman to a teenage Asian girl. "Want to squeeze the melons."

But I knew what she really wanted was to squeeze my butt cheeks. Why, I had no idea.

"Fuck off," I murmured.

A middle-aged Latino guy with a cowboy hat on said to a younger Latino guy, "Need a new hunting rifle to add to my collection." This was code for, *Gonna shoot me a mentally ill white guy,* who of course was me. My paranoia flared, and I wondered if he was packing a pistol on his other hip, where I couldn't see it from where I sat.

"Fuck off," I mumbled, a little louder.

Then two white teenagers started in on me. One held a skateboard, and he said to the other: "I hope we kick ass at the next game. Last one kind of sucked."

That was teen-speak for *Let's kick this old man's ass.* It was about me, naturally. It *all* was about me. My mind started to spin, and I felt weak and vulnerable. I couldn't take on the whole bus. All these people were about to beat the hell out of me, and the bus driver would probably urge them to greater violence. A hallucination flashed, of me nailed to a cross and set on fire.

It was the end; I was doomed.

A young woman held a toddler in her lap. The little boy was maybe two years old, not really old enough to speak, but he turned his head toward me and smiled and cooed a little bit.

All of a sudden I knew he was on my side. He was my only ally. I felt such a rush of relief that I nearly wept.

The toddler clapped his hands together and smiled, and everyone on the bus shut up. There were no more attacks, no more veiled threats, no more burning crosses. The little boy, to celebrate his victory, sat down in his mother's lap and promptly went to sleep.

Countdown voices became louder. They weren't there all the time, but several times a day they came back and did their thing.

"976, 42, 975, 974, 973, 41…" Countdown to violence, or countdown to involuntary confinement in the bug house? As the days dragged on, the numbers became lower and lower.

I became angry that I had so little control over my own life. I sent pissed-off emails to friends and was perturbed when I called my family. I accused them of working with Heather to keep me mentally ill. It had been years since things had been this bad, and everyone told me to stay on my meds and stick it out.

Gritting it out meant putting up with the harassment at my volunteer time at the library. The minor voices continued sounding off with numbers even there, and they made lewd comments about the books I was reading and the people who visited the art gallery.

After a few volunteer stints that were basically long attacks on my character, I decided that if this down cycle didn't end soon, I'd have to give up volunteering. It seemed to me that the patrons who came into the gallery caused the voices to begin with. Even if the patrons just asked what was on exhibit, or who managed the gallery, more noise filled my head. It was worse than at the café, because I was only at the café about an hour, and I was at the library for two hours. So the symptoms had time to build on themselves.

Maybe in response to continuing to volunteer at the library, the voices amped up their attacks. I called my shrink and complained. She upped my dose of Risperidone and told me to watch out for side effects, especially tremors in my hands and feet. There was nothing else she could do.

I had endless paranoid fantasies about the police attacking me, killing me, locking me up, crippling me, and so forth, and politicians using the police to get me. These delusions alternated with Heather howling in my ear that she was coming from L.A. to personally see to it I gave her some children. She was bringing LAPD cops to see that everything went her way. Between threats of police violence and worries about side effects from the medicines I took, I had meltdowns every couple days. I would just lay on my bed with the pillow over my head, almost unable to function. Every time a police car went by, my anxiety spiked. Every day or two I went to the Greyhound web site and looked up tickets, sometimes to Los Angeles and sometimes to Santa Fe, New Mexico.

The bursts of anger became intense, with frequent attacks throughout the day. I had to get Heather. I had to do something bad to her. Kill her. I had to stop her from these constant assaults on my sanity.

But how could I do that? How could I attack a voice in my head? Heather was just a vicious symptom stuck in my psyche. The only thing I could hope to do was outrun her.

If I had been in my right mind, I would have known this was a losing strategy. In 2007 and 2008 I had tried to outrun the voices all the way from Wisconsin to Egypt to Santa Fe. Heather and the minor voices had held on through several changes of medicine, several months of psychotherapy, and the attempts of friends and family to shake me loose from my symptoms by staying touch and offering their own voices instead of the mentally ill voices. The voices had held on for nine years, through all those changes and counter-attacks, and it would be a cinch for them to hang on through a move to Santa Fe.

Heather weighed in: "Are you going to *visit* Santa Fe, or *move* there? Which is it?" As she spoke, a police SWAT van, oversized and painted black, pulled up in front of my building. The back doors of the van opened, and ten very large men in black helmets and body armor hustled out. They were armed with shields and M-4 assault rifles. They brought with them several huge German Shepherds also dressed in body armor. These men surged up the steps of the building to reach the door, which Heather opened for them.

"Meet my friends," she snickered. "They're here to straighten you out."

I stopped listening to her and waited for heavy steps on the stairs. The cops were silent. Even their K-9's didn't bark.

It took a minute, but I summoned my courage and opened my front door. There was not a single cop to be seen.

Heather didn't say a thing. She stood there, off to one corner of my vision, and let me contemplate what this delusion meant. It was as clear a threat as I could ever imagine. I had three choices: find Heather in Los Angeles; go head to head with the police, or run.

I got on the computer and bought bus tickets to Albuquerque. Fueled by terror, I printed out the tickets and set them on my desk. It took no more than twenty minutes to pack a small backpack. I took only bare essentials: my medicines, a sleeping bag, a few changes of clothes, some empty plastic bottles for water, my checkbook for paying the rent on my room should I stay in Santa Fe into November, and a few postage stamps. I then spent a sleepless night of high anxiety, worrying about the many things that could go wrong. I wasn't acting on a plan, I was acting on emotion. A down cycle could go on for half a year or longer. I just didn't have what it took to live with this level of illness for so long a time. I'd done it before, out of necessity, but I was sure I couldn't do it again.

The bus ride to Albuquerque was long, nineteen hours, and frequently on the way Heather showed up in my head.

"Run, little rabbit, run!" she howled gleefully. "Where will you leave us behind—Phoenix? Flagstaff? Where?"

I sat in the seat, eating salted peanuts, and long before I reached Phoenix I realized I probably wasn't going to ditch her. My anger receded, and the terror grew stronger. But I was determined to *try* to get rid of her. I had to do *something*. It was hideous, trying to live my life in San Diego with unceasing interference.

Heather cackled again in Flagstaff, and the minor voices threw buzzwords into my mind. One of the minor voices said, "We know your future. We know the *real* story of your life. It's all laid out according to plan. All you've done with this bus ride is waste a pile of money. *Loser.*"

In Albuquerque I got off the bus with my bag and got onto the Rail Runner train that took me to Santa Fe. The trip was uneventful, and I actually enjoyed riding up into the mountains.

The air in Santa Fe felt chilly, so I put on a light jacket and trudged along the streets. In half an hour I arrived at the cement culvert where I had spent a month as a homeless person, back in 2008. There was a lot more graffiti on the bridge over the culvert, and more colorful graffiti. My biggest fear was that other homeless people had moved into the culvert, but as I checked out the situation, there was no one there but me. I dropped my bag onto the concrete and walked to the library. There was a big dumpster outside the La Farge Library, and I dug around in this and got a large cardboard box, which I broke down and then put in the tunnel, to sleep on. So began my second episode of living with mental illness in Santa Fe.

Time was not divided into discrete days. When I was hungry, I went to a nearby grocery store and bought a can of soup. When I was tired, I slept. Sometimes I walked around in random patterns, as the voices in my head guided me according to their whims.

"You're in Santa Fe," noted Heather, the day after I moved in under the bridge.

Immediately I felt God-awful. My guts hurt, my heart was full of pain, and I felt spin-headed. I hadn't ditched her. I hadn't outrun the torment. I had gone almost a thousand miles, spent hundreds of dollars, and invested days of my life in an effort to outrun the voices, and Heather was still there.

"Let's play a game," she said brightly.

I looked around but couldn't see her anywhere; she was just a voice in my head. A sense of foreboding came over me.

She cleared her throat and said, "My game is called, 'where are the cops?'"

I knew that somewhere, she was smiling.

"I think the cops in San Diego notified the cops in Santa Fe that you were coming. Expect company, any day now. I *told* you to go to Los Angeles, but here you are in New Mexico. I think the cops should knee-cap you, as punishment. At the very least."

I waited, teeth gritted, and she went away. She was satisfied; she had delivered her threat.

At least once a day I walked past the Life Link, which is the treatment facility that took me in when I was homeless and raving, and stabilized my condition, back in 2008. But every time I went past, it felt wrong to go inside. I did not want to revisit the past. I wanted to move on in the present. I wanted an end to schizoaffective disorder.

"What do you think of my game?" she asked, almost purring.

I can wait for weeks, maybe months. I can outlast you, Heather.

"Fuck nut, you've been trying to outlast me for almost a decade," she laughed. "You think a little change of scenery is going to beat me? Get on the bus. Go to Los Angeles. Do it. NOW."

I got up and started toward the library, but night had fallen, and I knew the library was closed. I went back into the tunnel and unrolled my sleeping bag and got inside. She babbled at me all night.

The voices became stronger and started a new game.

"Let's play 'elimination,'" said a voice. These were the little voices, which didn't have distinct personalities, like Heather did. I couldn't tell the minor voices apart. There were half a dozen of these lurking around.

Fuck you, I thought.

"Here's how you play, for example: the Life Link."

Memories of my seven months in The Life Link treatment center shot through my mind. I had flashbacks of the psychiatrist who prescribed my medicines, and the social workers who handled my case and helped me get my benefits rolling. I thought of my apartment and the communal meals that all of us sickos made for the holidays. These were pleasant memories, and suddenly they were gone. I felt bereaved, as though I had lost something precious.

"Let's do another one," said the voice. "Your books." I thought of my small collection of books back in San Diego, and I felt an acute pain in my heart. I had brought a few books with me to Santa Fe, but I could not really concentrate on reading them, with all the noise in my head. I felt certain that I had never written a book of my own, in my whole life. The voices insisted I had stolen e-books on the internet and put my name on them. That made me a criminal, and the cops would punish me. Then, just like that, I could no longer remember any books. Not books I had written, not books I had read. They were just gone.

"Easy game, huh?" said the voice. "Parents." Misery settled in as I thought of my father's bouts with cancer. Every day was a fight. He talked sometimes of beating the disease, and my mother emphasized that he wasn't getting worse, but he wasn't getting better, either. Cancer was murderous, and it had set its sights on my dad.

After a moment my father faded from my mind, and all the grim memories of his cancer battles went away.

"Hey," said a different voice. "Here's one: pistol."

And now I had a memory of the incident in Las Vegas, where I had almost murdered 40 people, back in early 2008. This vision horrified me, and this time I was the one who backed away from it. It was an old memory that wasn't as strong as more recent material, and in a few seconds it faded. It would be many months before I would be able to explore this incident dispassionately. For now it was just a bargaining chip the voices could play against me.

All that day words and phrases burned through my mind. Memories of various events from my mentally ill life fired, and I experienced misery, sorrow, pain, shock. I felt a lot of anger directed toward the voices. I fought off these negative feelings over and over again. Sometimes I was forced to wallow in them for hours. It was hard to sleep, and I became disheveled and crabby.

After a few days under the bridge, one of the voices took my side. It said, "Do you want these attacks to stop?"

Of course, I thought.

"Give your friend Jackie a command word, 'turquoise.' This is a gift from the American Indians. Your friend can make the voices stop. Do it today or tomorrow; this is a limited time offer."

Days melted together like colors on a bad painting; I walked around downtown Santa Fe and even visited some of the museums. The memories that had disappeared during our game of elimination came back. I sent an email to my friend Jackie, and in the middle of the email I typed 'turquoise' with no explanation of what it meant. She replied to the email but didn't address the word. I waited anxiously to see what would happen, and another day went by.

Of course, the voices did not quit. They did not even slow down a little bit. They bit at me night and day, constantly, and I was in shock. The voices had, in 2008, pointed me to Santa Fe to begin with, and there I had found help for my illness. Now, seven years later, I had really believed that typing 'turquoise' in an email to a friend would shut the voices down.

Heather laughed at my reaction. "You stupid fuck," she giggled. I couldn't see her, but she was close. I knew that much. "We test you constantly, to see if you're listening. Dumb ass. One little word isn't going to do a thing, but maybe if you obey us for *fifty* command words, we'll help you out."

'What is the point of 'elimination'?" I asked.

"When we've absorbed all your memories, and taken over your whole brain, then we'll let you go," she sneered.

Now I was just confused, because the voices gave conflicting information. Respond to command words, and be set free. Play 'elimination' to its conclusion, and be set free. Find the real story behind 9/11 and find my destiny.

"Or come to L.A. and knock me up. I'll help you get a job, and you can support me," said Heather. "That'll be the new free."

I lay on my sleeping bag in the tunnel (this was at night, and I couldn't sleep), and I said to her: "The command word didn't work. You're lying. All the voices are lying."

"Papa tower, mama tower, baby tower. Who is lying?" Her voice crackled with energy. "Three baby towers is what I want. I really don't care what *you* want."

Her voice faded away.

Somewhere around then the voices changed their tune. It wasn't Heather but some minor voice which said, in the early morning hours as I walked to Denny's for breakfast: "Let's talk about what's *really* going on in your life. We've told you that you're worth a hundred million dollars, and that's nice, but did you know you're famous around the globe?"

"Heather said something about my stories being published in 70 languages," I murmured. I had bought into this and believed it.

"Your accomplishments go deeper than just publishing some

stories and making money," the voice hummed. "Hollywood has little cameras everywhere you go. There are cameras in the culvert where you sleep, and cameras in the grocery store, and cameras in your place in San Diego, and on and on. And we have machines in your eyeglasses, to read your mind. There is another machine in your sleeping bag, to read your thoughts when you're asleep."

This statement gave me the creeps. I was sure the voice was telling me the truth. I knew people in San Diego could read my mind, and I knew they could insert their own thoughts into my head.

"Why?" I asked.

"We want to know *all* about you," said the voice. "Every little detail. Hollywood and the music industry and the New York publishing people are slicing your life up into pieces and making art out of it. Pay attention, now! Here's how it works: the cameras and the microphones and the mind reading machines collect everything. Then a team of psychiatrists sorts it all out into categories, like 'thoughts about writing,' 'thoughts about reading,' 'thoughts about the cops,' 'ideas for fantasy stories,' 'ideas for science fiction,' and so forth. There are dozens of categories."

"I'm not that interesting," I said.

"That's because you don't know what we're doing with all that raw material. We're sorting it into categories and then licensing each idea, each incident, to an artist. So some Hollywood screenwriter might buy up an idea for a sci-fi screenplay. He'll throw a hundred dollars into your kitty, and develop the idea. If the screenplay actually makes it to production into a movie, the screenwriter will throw much more, like a thousand dollars, into your account. Same with books. Same with music. Guess what? This is *global.* Hundreds of thousands of artists around the globe are participating. That's where all your money is coming from."

As the voice said this, I couldn't help but feel amazed. This was so huge and so deep. "When do I meet these people?"

"You'll meet some of the key players in due time. You may

actually be worth more than a hundred million; the numbers change constantly."

"So I'm a world-famous writer. All the pieces are falling into place," I babbled. I felt a burst of excitement, and I continued: "I really want to meet these people. It must be an incredible project."

"Every week there is a five-minute video that your handlers in Hollywood post to the web," the voice said with confidence. "It has the highlights of your past week. Somewhere along the way, some politicians got on board. They started commenting with jokes and riddles and funny sayings about you. People liked this and asked for more. I won't bore you with details, but let's just say, what ended up happening is that the politicians, in other countries as well as here, started feeling sorry for you. It was obvious that you were tormented by voices and crippled by paranoia, and brought down by attacks of irrational fear.

"Something good came out of all this misery. The leaders of Israel and the Palestinian people watched you suffer for years, laughing at your exploits as your illness made a hash of your life. They then realized that the joke was on them. Here you were, crippled and half-dead, and you were making efforts to better yourself. Meanwhile, they were looking to kill each other."

"This is a lot of information," I said, starting to get a headache.

"Want me to make a long story short?" said the voice, annoyed.

"Please. It's hard to concentrate."

"You're going to receive the Nobel Peace Prize. Israel and the Palestinians got it together and made peace. They cited you as their inspiration."

I had breakfast at Denny's, as the voices gibbered on about nothing. Then I walked back to the tunnel, and in a few hours the library opened. I got on a computer and went to the Nobel Prize web site, where there was a list of the year's winners. My name was not there.

Immediately a voice (same voice, or different? who could tell?)

said, "Next year's list. They publish in October. Look for the prize next year. Remember, all these prize winners had to wait years to be recognized. You've got more commendations on the way, too."

"Like what? More 'inspiration' stuff?"

"That's enough for today. Just stumble around like an idiot, and we'll make a video of your miseries. You're saving the world from itself, old man, all due to a handful of media elites and a great idea."

"Sounds kind of like *The Truman Show,* but with a political slant," I grumbled.

"We'll tell you about China later."

All this sounded promising, and exciting, and I wondered why I was still homeless and sick in the head when these voices told me my bank account was stuffed full of money, and I was ten years younger than I thought I was.

The next day, the countdown voices returned: "954, 953, 87, 86, 952…" They went on and on, and I had a deep fear that if the cops caught me under the bridge, I'd be thrown in jail.

A couple of days went by. From time to time I went to the La Farge library and sent emails to friends, trying to keep up a façade of normalcy. I told no one that I was in Santa Fe, or why I went there.

The voices kept up their chatter, playing games and threatening to sic the police on me. Every day I had a strong urge to flee. Flee anywhere. Go somewhere I had not been before or had not been for a long time. This was just like the urge to get out of San Diego, and I didn't trust this instinct, this time. Running to Santa Fe had cost me a couple hundred dollars, and nothing had improved. Could I escape the voices in my head if I ran far, far away?

Then a lone voice came into my mind. I am not sure if this was during morning, day, or night. The hours of the day had a way of blurring together, and the voices gibbered one after the next, so that what happened in the world mixed with what happened in my head.

"You are due for more awards," bleated the voice. This one was not Heather, either; just a minor voice, a nobody among voices.

"Fuck off," I mumbled.

The voice hissed. "You better hear me out. Are you listening?"

"Fuck you." I tried to will the voice away, but that didn't work.

"CHINA IS PULLING OUT OF TIBET," said the voice. "Because of *you*. Because it's *funny* to watch some mentally ill asswipe run around with his hands on his head, whispering 'fuck off' all the time, unable to tell reality from delusion."

Misery washed over me. The voices were just getting started with me. Good God, why wasn't the increased dose of medicine working?

"Loser," said the voice. "Haven't you always known we're stronger than the medicine?"

"GO AWAY," I yelled. I was in my sleeping bag in the cement tunnel; the sky was dark. Vaguely I worried that someone was walking over the tunnel and would hear me and call the police.

"The President of China is a big fan of your videos," said the voice. "He really likes it when you get crazy urges to travel. He said that this is like the crazy ideas his subordinates get, and then they try to convince him to follow them."

"Someone is filming me in the tunnel?" I croaked feebly. I knew I was being recorded, video and audio, but the thought that I was *this* vulnerable was frightening. "When is all this going to *stop*?"

"The President of the United States is going to award you with the Presidential Medal of Freedom with distinction, for the incredible strides you've made for global peace."

I concentrated on breathing in and breathing out. I could see this medal in a frame, in my room in San Diego. I could see the Nobel Peace Prize right alongside it.

The voice went on: "The Queen of England wants to knight you. Knighthood! Anytime you're ready! All this is yours, just for a little unhappiness… Stand tall. Stand proud. Fight hard. Be loud!"

"Videos?" I croaked.

"That's just technical stuff," said the voice. "You want to know how the system works? YOU created the system. It was YOUR idea. Every week we post a short video highlighting your latest symptoms. And people watch it. For countries with poor internet access, we put the video on television, or run a few still photos in the national newspapers. You're everywhere!"

"So what?" I said. A part of me, a big part, was screaming right then, trying to break free of delusions and psychosis and schizoaffective disorder. But my attempt to escape didn't work, and I remained a prisoner in my own skull.

"They make pledges. The heads of state, the CEO's of major corporations, five star generals of the world's military forces, and so on and so forth. They pledge to convert to green energy. They pledge large sums of money to building new schools and new hospitals. They pledge to reduce the size of standing armies; that is, they commit to ten years of peace. See the pattern? While we torture you with ten years of suffering, the world enjoys a decade of peace. It's a direct relationship.

"And those leaders, they submit 'hits' against you. The President of China, for instance, wants you to hear four hours of bad Chinese music. That's in return for pulling the Chinese military out of Tibet. It's all interconnected. You're at the center of the largest social/artistic/political/military/educational/peace/love/business movement in history. Everyone is getting in on it.

"They're all making pledges. Leaders are ending wars and calling the soldiers home. Governments are putting up money to fight diseases. REAL money. And if some country's leaders don't have enough cash to make a strong pledge, the Europeans and Americans are giving big grants. It's all about YOU, guy. One man serving as the inspiration to save the whole world."

Then the voice went away.

I lay there in my sleeping bag and let all this surge through my mind. The idea was plausible. Certainly there were great people in history who had an incredible impact on millions and even billions of lives. People like Genghis Khan, and Robert Oppenheimer and Jonas Salk. People like Mohammed and Jesus and the Buddha.

Clearly I was no great man myself. Look at me: broken down and not only poor but deep in debt, my head full of weird voices and crazy thoughts and strange urges to run and run away...

But as a warning to others, an inspiration of what *not* to become, maybe I had a little value. The bonfire of psychosis was a flame that lit up the whole world.

It was so clear to me that this explanation was pure crazy, but I believed it. The idea was so bizarre, so illuminating, that I could see the world's leaders going for it.

Five or six days into my stay in Santa Fe—this was in the sunny afternoon—three city workers came to my tunnel and stood in the canyon that the tunnel fed into. They talked for twenty minutes about work they were going to do in the canyon. This would take several weeks and would be noisy. There would be people and machines in the canyon.

There was no way I could stay in my tunnel. The workers were going to begin their project in a few days, and I had to find another place. I roamed around the area, looking for a circle of bushes I could hide in, or something similar. I found more culverts in the area, but they both had puddles in them, so that was no good. Then I went a little farther away and found a small culvert with some dead branches for cover. It took a while, but I moved all my stuff there and prepared to be cramped.

A few days went by, and the urge to flee became stronger and stronger. Every morning I bolted from the culvert and practically ran to the grocery store to get something for breakfast. I went to the library every day and looked at bus ticket prices to New York City, Salt Lake City, San Diego, and of course Los Angeles. The price tags were in the hundreds of dollars, one-way. L. A., really? Right to Heather?

I looked up the weather forecast for Salt Lake City and realized it was heading for winter in the mountains. Cold temperatures and frost. I was not prepared for that kind of weather. I would have to spend more money on insulated socks, a better pair of shoes/boots, thick clothes, and a winter coat…

It seemed smarter not to commit to any destination but to wait for a sign, like the voices pointing me to one city or another. Accordingly, I spent hours looking up maps of these four cities, printing off street maps of downtown and the area around the bus stations. I looked at temperature charts and maps with soup kitchens indicated on them. Maps with homeless shelters were next.

During the time I pursued these maps, the urge to run was so strong that I could hardly pay attention to what I did. I would print off a couple of maps and then abandon the computer and speed-walk to the grocery store, to buy some apples to eat. Then I would head back to the library, only to find that the librarian had given the computer to someone else, and I had to wait forty-five minutes for the next available computer.

The pressure built, and about halfway through October I sat in front of a computer. Clearly I could survive in any of the four cities I was thinking of. I knew where the homeless shelters were, and the soup kitchens. But which city to run to?

"You *know* which city," said Heather in an ugly tone of voice.

I responded by taking a quarter out of my pocket and thinking, *heads: New York City, and tails: Salt Lake City.* I flipped the coin into the air and caught it: Salt Lake City. *heads: Salt Lake City; tails: San Diego.* Flip. Salt Lake City. *heads: Salt Lake City; tails: Los Angeles.* Flip. The coin spun in the air half a dozen times, and I missed it when I tried to catch it. It fell on the computer desk and made a loud clinking sound. It was tails. I was going to Los Angeles.

Heather just smiled.

I bought the ticket and printed it off and shoved it in my pocket, and then I searched for hotels near the LA bus station. I felt ill; this move, determined wholly by chance, was sending me straight into the lion's den. Even Lady Luck answered to Heather.

The next day I was on my way. Not once had I gone to the Life Link, the whole week I was living in the culverts. My visit to Santa Fe was just an expensive way of failing; the voices had not stopped or even slowed down. If anything, they had revealed more layers of delusion, and I was sicker than ever.

It took about twenty hours to get to Los Angeles, and Heather was with me most of the time, laughing and slapping her hands on her knees. She was extremely pleased. I kept wondering if she had rigged the coin toss somehow. Not by manipulating the coin itself, but my manipulating what I *thought* I saw. Certainly I would be foolish not to entertain the possibility.

"Whooo-eeee, fuck head, come to MY city! Forget those hicks in Santa Fe! Come to the center of the universe!"

I couldn't remember if I had ever seen this side to her. She usually was happy only if I was miserable. This seemed like surefire proof that there really was a vast conspiracy. The voice of Heather wasn't in my head; it was in a tiny nano-speaker embedded in the collar of my shirt. Maybe the speaker was in one arm of my eyeglasses, and Heather was some actress who represented Hollywood. It took Silicon Valley high tech and a Hollywood actress to tell these stories about my life, and to keep me running.

"What is your address?" I mumbled to her.

"No way, douche bag. You have to look for me! Find a hotel and drop your stuff, and start searching!"

Not long after this, the bus reached Los Angeles, and I got out. I went to a taxicab and told the driver the address of the nearest cheap hotel, and when we arrived I paid him. It took only a few minutes to check into the hotel, and then I started my deal with the devil.

I walked all over the neighborhood where the hotel was, and it didn't take me long to figure out that this area was heavily Latino.

"Where the fuck *are* you?" I asked Heather, who was appearing and disappearing in my mind as I walked along.

"You're getting colder," she said, as I stumbled around.

I searched for a couple hours, mostly going in circles. There were people on the street, but no red-haired white woman.

"This is nuts," I complained. "There must be a hundred neighborhoods in L.A., and millions and millions of people. There is no way I will find you, just walking around." It was like my mind had split in half. Half of me believed in Heather, that she would lead me to find her, and half of me knew this "search" was pure lunacy. These halves fought constantly, so sometimes I was angry as I walked along in the snipe hunt, because I knew I was not going to find anyone important, and sometimes I went along with it and stared at all the women I came across, because I thought it would be a real surprise if I did find Heather.

Around seven in the evening I went to a Mexican restaurant and ordered dinner.

"You didn't look very hard," Heather scolded me. "What's a couple of hours spent searching, in return for all I can give you?"

"Couple hours, you say," I mumbled. "You've been pushing me for nine years. I suppose I would like to meet you in person, but I'm not going to spend months wandering around L.A., looking for you."

"Did I ask you to?" she snapped. "DID I ASK YOU TO SPEND MONTHS SEARCHING FOR ME? FUCKWIT! Maybe a few weeks, a month. Be clever. Be smart. Be humble. You never try to ingratiate yourself to me. Suck up a little."

She went on for the whole meal, like: "You're half a man; only half of you believes in me, and that's the better half. The skeptic needs to die. Step out in traffic. Step in front of a bus. We'll get rid of Bad Randal and keep Good Randal." Then she ranted and raved and became incoherent.

I finished the food, paid for the meal, and returned to my hotel room. The day's travels had worn me out, and I took a shower and went to bed.

As soon as I woke the next morning, Heather said, "Hunt for me, or I'll scream all day."

This seemed like something she could really do, so I got out of bed and dressed and took another walk around the neighborhood. There was a little eatery where I had something for breakfast, and then I roamed far and wide and looked for my imaginary girlfriend. If Heather was here, she would have a hard time hiding. In the visual hallucinations I had about her, her hair was auburn. All I had to do was stop on a street corner and look up and down the streets, and I'd see her if she was within a few blocks.

"Can't you give me a hint?" I said in frustration. This was on the street; I wasn't even trying to keep my mouth shut. There weren't enough people around to hear me talk with an imaginary girlfriend.

"You're completely cold right now," she cooed. "You're not even in the right part of the city." Then she shut up.

This made me angry, and I stomped back through the streets to my hotel and got my pack. A minute later I was at the front office, where I asked the middle-age clerk to phone a taxi. I handed him the room key.

"Did you have a good stay?" he asked.

This made me even angrier, but I nodded and said, "The room was great. Having problems with my girlfriend."

Wisely, he didn't dig deeper. Instead he called the taxi, and I went outside and stood in front of the building. In a surprisingly short time the taxi came and took me to the Greyhound station.

I was supposed to meet with some other writers in San Diego that very day, to discuss the stories we were working on, but I knew I would not make the meeting. This failed get-together was just another casualty of mental illness.

The ticket from L.A. to San Diego was cheap, and in a few hours I was back in my own room in San Diego.

I had accomplished nothing of value; all I had done was waste about seven hundred dollars on food and transportation. It seemed incredible that Heather could take such control that she could urge me to go thousands of miles and spend money on things I *knew* I could not afford. It was going to take months to pay off the credit card debt, and what would happen if Heather gained the upper hand again and took me off on another spending spree?

A few days later, during my usual morning hour at the café, she seemed contrite as she said, "Don't you want a girlfriend?"

The implications of this were so grotesque that I could not even think of a response. An imaginary girlfriend who ran me down and threatened to push me to suicide, who forced her agenda on me all the time, and who urged me to all sorts of stupid acts.

"You're an asshole, you know that?" she barked. "I've been with you all these years, keeping you company and looking out for your best interests. You never say thank you, and you've never given me even one little kid. You wouldn't even know it's actually 2005, unless I tell you. You've got your whole life ahead of you, and it's filled with good stuff. And you wouldn't even go for it, up in L.A. You gave up in ONE day. What a fuck wad."

I took my morning walk, and then the minor voices came after me, when I was checking my email at home.

"Look on CNN's web site," said one voice. "They're talking about you."

Another voice said, "Your email account has a little tracker to see whose emails you open first, so we can tell who your most important friends are."

"Send an email to all your closest friends," said a third voice. "Put the command word, 'loser,' in the subject line."

This went on and on and was crippling; I could not read emails with all this noise in my head. Every time I changed web sites, the voices yelled suggestions and commands.

"GO TO PBS, OR I'LL FUCK YOU UP," a voice threatened.

"Get into your bank account, and send some money to the Queen of England. In fact, send ALL your money to her."

"Wouldn't you like a rare book? Look for one that costs a thousand dollars. Something in a language you don't speak or read."

These voices hounded me for several days. Sometimes I was able to push them aside and use my computer as I saw fit, and sometimes the voices had me going to all sorts of websites I wouldn't have visited on my own. Many of these were sites of artists, or talk about artists, or psychiatrists talking about the psychology of artists. That led me to sites about mental illness and creativity. You'd think I learned something useful from these sources, but I wasn't there because I wanted to learn. I was there because I lost battles with the voices, and they sent me to these web sites. So I clicked around, glanced at some images, read a few sentences, and then tried to return to the sites I wanted to read.

My life became a series of running fights. The voices played 'elimination.' They played 'buzzword bingo.' I saw the twin towers fall and remembered Heather's assertion that 9/11 was a fraud.

Thinking about Heather seemed to summon her:

"I told you about the pledges people are making," she said. "Well, the Prime Minister of India just abolished the remnants of the caste system, and has pledged billions of rupees to educate the poor. What did I say? Real progress! That's *you*, moron. You stagger around like a fool, accomplishing nothing, while world leaders accomplish great things. You're everyone's favorite fuck-up!"

I sent emails to friends, telling them about my hallucinations and delusions, and they asked if I was taking my meds. I was, but that was just another battle: meds or voices, which would win? I was on a low dose of Risperidone a day, and even that that caused my hands and feet to shake. My psychiatrist told me that this shaking can become permanent if you take the drug for a long time. This made me think of a friend of mine who suffered from bipolar disorder; his hands shook constantly from the medicines he was on. My tremors weren't nearly so bad as his, and so I stuck with the drug.

Because of my symptoms, sticking with my daily routine was difficult, but I stuck with my schedule out of sheer stubbornness and because my daily rounds were an anchor that allowed me to fight the voices. In the café I sort of scanned the pages of books, determined to get some pleasure out of them, but usually it was a long series of attacks from the voices, and I had to read and then re-read the words. But damn it, I managed to read a book here and there, and this gave me a sense of accomplishment that led to confidence to fight.

"Remember when we said you're worth a hundred million dollars?" Heather cajoled. "You're not. You're worth five *billion* dollars. They're taking up collections for you, all over the world. You're bigger than JFK, boyfriend. You're bigger than Gandhi, more important than MLK Jr., twice as relevant as Mandela. It's all about YOU, and you have to PAY to play!"

I went online and looked up 'what are the symptoms of schizoaffective disorder?' I found a whole laundry list, including this:

> **delusions of grandeur** - a delusion (common in paranoia) that you are much greater and more powerful and influential than you really are (online source: the Free Dictionary)

It seemed like virtually everything I thought I saw or had thoughts about was a symptom of mental illness. Where did schizoaffective disorder end and normalcy begin? Was it 'normal' to read a book, when voices constantly interrupted? Could it be said I took a walk, when every step was filled with Heather babbling on about how the President of the United States had scrapped the entire nuclear arms stockpile, and every other nuclear-armed nation on earth had followed suit, because of me? Was I really typing emails to friends, when the words were dictated by little voices in my head? Sometimes I belonged to myself, and sometimes the voices had me.

"College is now free in the U.S.," Heather said, breathlessly. This was near the end of October. I looked forward to Halloween, but Heather only wanted to spin out more delusions. I was on my computer, reading emails from friends, and she was trying to harass me with more warped thinking.

I stopped reading emails and went to a search engine and typed in, 'is college free in the United States?' Results came back, I scanned a few pages, and Heather laughed.

"You believe those guys, but you don't believe me?" she tittered.

"This stuff you're telling me, it's not real," I said through gritted teeth. "IT'S NOT REAL."

So she waited until I went back to my friends' emails and got engrossed in what they were saying, and then she whispered, "Free college isn't going on right away. It's going to take the schools a year or two to get the system worked out. The citizens of the U.S. put it to a vote, and they overwhelmingly voted for free college for any citizen who passed the entrance exams."

And I believed her. It came down to who was there the most often, some journalist or pundit on a web site, or Heather and her minor voice friends, whispering away day and night. I didn't like Heather; she never acted in my best interests. But she was there almost *every* day, and she knew me very, very well. She knew which buttons to push, what to say and how to say it, to build her version of reality.

I fought her. Lord, did I fight. Back in 2014 some VA psychologists offered me classes on Cognitive Behavioral Social Skills Training (CBSST). I took the classes and learned some techniques for fighting Heather and the other voices, and battling the paranoia and delusions. When she told me lies, I whispered the truth. When she threatened to sic the cops on me, I said, "Where are they? Bring them on." But my efforts were not terribly effective, and in general, by the time I became aware of her attacks, she had already convinced me to believe her. It's like an enemy army taking over 75% of your country, and at that point you think, *Maybe I should fight back?* But by that time most of your army has been subverted, and the rest have only bb guns to fight with.

"I want three kids," she said. Every. Single. Day. "Come to Los Angeles and help me with my career."

"I went to Los Angeles. I couldn't find you. That adventure cost me $800. Now go away."

She gave a shrieking laugh. "That's just the beginning! You need to go to San Francisco, your old stomping grounds. Go now, and spend a week looking around. Halloween is always so much fun there! San Francisco! Now!"

I had a very strong urge to go to San Francisco, and I had to fight like hell not to buy a ticket. I went to my credit card statement and stared at my debts, and the cold, hard reality of the numbers allowed me to ignore her.

After a while she said, "Give me three kids. Jerk off into an envelope, and send it to me. I'll do the rest."

Somehow I managed not to respond to this, and she went away.

So here is what it was like, Halloween evening at my favorite café:

Heather: "When do the freaks come out?"

Me: *Look around! There's a guy dressed up like Thor, right across the street.*

Heather: "They should dress up like me. I'm a character."

Minor Voice 1: "Let's play elimination. 'Masters degree.'" Sure as hell, I thought of my classes, professors, and diploma, and then it all disappeared from my mind.

Minor Voice 2: "'Years in the Army.'" I thought of some of the men I knew during my enlistment in the military, back in my twenties, and then those experiences were gone.

In the café, someone's cell phone rang. This was one of the other patrons in the café, and in my delusional state, a ringing phone meant that whoever was talking in my head was getting support from the person on the phone. The phone fed Heather and her friends.

The minor voices shut up for a while. I watched ghosts, witches, body builders, Captain America, and a bloody murder victim walk down the sidewalk outside the café.

Minor Voice 1: "khamsa" We were switching from elimination to buzzword bingo.

Minor Voice 2: "everything" Meaning, we were going to review absolutely every thing that had ever happened to me. Accordingly, I had flashbacks to earlier parts of my life. Memories cascaded through my mind, and the people in costumes celebrating Halloween became people from my childhood, when I went trick-or-treating. These images only lasted seconds, and then they disappeared.

Minor Voice 3: "perfect" When we had reviewed all my memories and gotten rid of the irrelevant ones, I would be perfect.

Minor Voice 4: "heaven" It's heaven with Heather.

Heather: "Mother fucker. Why won't you go to San Francisco? It's nice there this time of year. Nice and cool, rainy. Come to meet me. I'll guide your way. It's not *that* costly."

Me: "It's more than I can afford. Tell you what. You come to me. You know where I live. You can—"

Heather: "Stupid ass. *You* follow *me*, not the other way around. Get on a fucking bus and go to San Francisco. Better yet, fly."

So I spent my Halloween night, until Heather ran out of steam.

And on that note, I cruised unhappily into November.

November: delusions

In November the weather became noticeably cooler, quite nice after the summer heat. My father tried to hang tough in his battle against cancer, but my mother said he was weak from the chemo.

"The oncologist told us that melanoma is a very aggressive cancer," she said on the phone. "For now we have it under control, but it *will* come back. That's what he said. Not 'maybe' or 'could,' but 'almost certainly will.'"

"Heather is like a cancer, too," I said miserably. "She drives out the good thoughts with her poison, and she takes over."

There was a long pause on the phone.

"Can't you get your psychiatrist to give you more powerful medicine?" she asked.

"Side effects get really bad, if I do that," I said. "I guess it's heartening to know dad is sticking in there."

"Here he is; talk to him yourself."

My dad got on the phone. "Yeah, I'm okay. Your mother worries too much." He sounded tired and weak.

"Are you going deer hunting with your brothers?" I asked him, because he did this almost every year.

Pause. "No, I'm not going to make it this year," he said. "Want to, but not well enough to even sit in a stand for a few hours. I get tired at every little exertion. Good to hear from you, and here's your mom back." He handed her the receiver.

"We're just taking it one day at a time," my mother said. "I really wish I had spotted that tumor before it got into his lymph nodes. Now we have to see what happens with the chemo. We're trying everything we can. I hope you and your brother never come down with this."

I almost said, "Heather will find a way to kill me before then," but I managed to censor this. "I'll say a prayer for both of you," I said, and then we hung up.

The progress of my father's cancer brought my spirits down. He had had cancer for several years by this point, and I was getting used to the treatments and general ill health that came from melanoma. There was nothing I could do to help him; even asking him to come to the phone to talk for a minute felt like I was punishing the old man. So my role in his cancer war was to offer good cheer and try to console him for all the things he had once enjoyed and could no longer do.

Because I was due to be rich and famous any day now, I went on the internet and looked for art that I could purchase to decorate the big Victorian house I intended to buy. I spent hours staring at paintings by Keith Parkinson and Larry Elmore, who do fantasy paintings featuring pretty women and hungry dragons. I picked my favorites and jotted down the names of the paintings I wanted to buy. I was *just* sane enough that I didn't actually try to purchase them; I knew I had to wait until the money came in before I closed the deal.

I spent more time looking up feather artists and came across a website featuring Beth McCormick, who makes stunning pieces of art out of masks and feathers, or feathers and fur. Again I picked my favorites, and this time I was so amazed that I sent an email and asked for quotes. A few days later she got back to me with a general range of prices. Needless to say, they were far, far beyond what I could actually afford.

Since everyone knew me, and I was famous for my stories and books, and virtually everyone on the planet watched my videos every week, I began to walk around with my chest pushed out, expecting someone to break the wall of false news that the media kept around me.

One afternoon in early November, as I took a walk on the Martin Luther King Jr. promenade, Heather said, "What are you doing, walking around looking for people to acknowledge your success?"

"What would you do, if you were the greatest man in all history but everyone pretended you were just some mentally ill loser?"

"I'd give Heather 3 kids, and move to Los Angeles to help her with her career."

I want my awards, I thought at her. There were other people on the promenade, and I couldn't have a conversation with her out loud.

"Act like you want it," she said. "Do what I tell you, and you'll get your prizes."

So running around LA like a dumb shit, looking for you, is a good idea?

"Name me a job where there are no unpleasant aspects," she said.

I either want my goodies, or I want you and the other voices out.

"Listen to you! Pay up or get out! How are you going to do that, fuck-mobile? Put a gun to your head and pull the trigger? That'll do it. How are those meds working for you? HUH?"

After that, she and the other voices went back to their usual messages, and I didn't challenge her again. I had been trying to get rid of her for years, and nothing worked. She was entrenched, and I was along for the ride.

The cops watched me. Every time I saw a black and white prowler cruise past, the car slowed down, and the driver and his partner eyed me up. This happened every few days. I was afraid to say anything to my friends or family about this situation, because they might side with the cops.

I knew the police were taking tips from Heather. She fed them all sorts of tidbits about me. She was going to convince the cops to bring false charges and put me away forever, and then she was going to claim I had married her and was due the full sum of my net worth. It was her against my family, or maybe they'd just split my money down the middle...

Going out of my room remained a fearful experience. I read something on the internet about computer hackers taking over the camera on your computer and watching you; I was sure this was happening to me.

Were the cops going to kill me, or were they only going to put me away for the rest of my life? How could I avoid them? I lived right in downtown San Diego, and police patrols were frequent. Worse yet, cops came into the café from time to time, to get a coffee or a snack. They walked right past me sometimes. My blood pressure spiked, and I watched their hands to see if they would pull a gun.

And the homeless people were in on it, too, because the cops paid them to snitch. On my daily walking route, I always encountered homeless people sleeping in doorways or on the sidewalk. That is, they *pretended* to sleep. In truth, they were videotaping me mumbling to myself.

Then I knew what was really going on: Heather was going to take *all* my money, and I was going to end up homeless. If I fought her, she'd have the cops blow me away. All the signs were there: I had been homeless before, and history ran in cycles that repeated themselves. I had been homeless back in 2007-2008, and I would almost certainly be homeless again. The cops would think it funnier if they reduced me to homelessness rather than to shoot me, which someone might raise an outcry from my community.

I spoke to a friend of mine, and he said he and his wife weren't going to invite me over for Thanksgiving dinner. They were going to visit his father, far away, for the holiday. So I had to make other arrangements for Turkey Day. I looked into it and found that history was indeed repeating itself; the Salvation Army was hosting its annual Thanksgiving Day dinner at Golden Hall, a short walk from my place. I had gone there before, and I would go there this year, too. The lady at the local Salvation Army office gave me a card with the location and time printed on it, and I was good to go.

The boundaries between reality and delusion became slippery. At the café, in the mornings, I noticed a number of people approaching me and sniffing at me, as if to suggest I reeked. Since I was only taking a shower every three or four days, and God only know how often I washed clothes, there was probably some truth to these thoughts.

But then one white-haired old man in a rain jacket stopped a few feet from me, and he took a deep sniff. This was at the café, where I was pouring half and half into my coffee.

He's sniffing up my thoughts, to report to Heather. I knew it without anyone having to tell me a thing. All these sniffers were her agents. She had the cops, the homeless, and random people at the café, all on her side.

The voices stopped hammering me ten hours a day and only came around an hour or two. They talked about 9/11 a lot, about the planes, the murdered Americans, and the hijackers.

"All fake," said a minor voice, as I worked on my novel, *Political Mommies.* "The attack on 9/11 was the point at which you lost track of reality and entered a fake world of media perception. We've told you this before. But you're going to win in all of this. Eventually it'll all work to your favor."

When? I howled at the voice. *This has been going on for years.*

"Be patient," said the voice.

Every so often a police car cruised by the café, or I saw the police Homeless Outreach Team van, and I knew these sightings were an implied threat. The cops were going to seize my belongings, and I'd become homeless. Sometimes, as I went on a nice walk for exercise, I would pass cops who were talking to the homeless, or talking to agitated citizens who shouted and threw out wild accusations against their neighbors, and so forth.

These events terrified me. Heather was putting cops in my face every few days. She was just daring me to say something, or start something. How could I fight all these forces arrayed against me?

As if to taunt me, the minor voices played aggressive games of elimination: "you don't have a masters degree; you dropped out of high school" "lived in San Francisco for twenty years? how can that be, it's only 2005?" "what do you mean, you served in the army? you don't have the balls to be a soldier" "*how* many books have you written? NONE! they're gibberish, every one of them. go back and read them: all work and no play makes Jack a dull boy"

I couldn't hold onto the details of my own past, and it seemed that all my accomplishments involved lies and half-truths. In desperation I went to my copies of the books I had written over my 30 years of writing, and they looked like garbage. It was like they were written by a chimpanzee randomly striking keys. I *knew* I had written them, but I emotionally speaking, they felt like someone else's cast-off garbage.

Heather came around every three or four days and repeated her demands for kids.

Once, as I was doing my daily writing and expecting Heather to show up, I saw a clear hallucination of my Uncle Ray in jungle green military uniform, Vietnam-era. This was one of my mother's brothers, and he had served in Vietnam. A lit cigarette hung out of his mouth, and he held an M-16 loosely in his hands. His hair was crew-cut, and he looked like a man just going into his old age. When I was a child he told me scary stories about fighting in the jungles of Vietnam, and in tunnels, and so forth.

"How you doing, Randy?" he asked. His eyes were on the rifle, not me.

I just stared. Full-on visual hallucinations were rare for me. "Fighting someone?" I asked him.

"She's coming. You know who. Gonna run her off. You can't see this; it's going to be ugly. Go on, now, go home."

And just like that I was back at my desk. I lost the visual hallucination, but the audio was turned up to full. Uncle Ray and Heather fought it out. For me this was most like a series of impulses, to beat up Heather, or to grab a pistol from Uncle Ray and see if I could kill Heather with it. I was deeply tired of my illness and willing to do damned near anything to get away from it.

The fight lasted a few minutes, and when it was over, Heather didn't show up. Uncle Ray said, "Showed *her* what's what," and the last thing I remember from that incident was Uncle Ray's cigarette smoke curling upward into the canopy foliage of Vietnam.

Uncle Ray slowed Heather down a bit, but two or three days later she retaliated while I took a shower: "Don't you want the money, at least? A billion dollars will buy a lot of art."

"Haven't I suffered enough?" I mumbled at her. "Years of this crap. And now it's bad again, and I can't tell when it will end."

"You haven't suffered. The Jews suffered, in Auschwitz. The Japanese-Americans suffered, in the internment camps. Talk to the American Indians, stuck on little chicken-shit reservations while the white people whoop it up on stolen land. Why don't you look this up: the Long Walk. The Trail of Tears. Go find out who Diego de Landa was. Yeah, religion is a *good* thing. Ha! Then come back to me and whine about how *you've* suffered."

This shamed me into silence.

By the middle of the month the voices were yammering on day and night. I could hardly sleep, and the meds didn't seem as strong as Heather and her friends. I had learned Cognitive Behavioral Social Skills Training (CBSST) techniques from a team of psychologists at the VA hospital, and I tried these techniques (which basically teach you to refocus your mind when your symptoms are attacking), but these didn't help much when the attacks were constant. I was afraid of the cops and afraid of the voices and afraid of the homeless people. I was even afraid of the sniffers, because they could strike me anywhere, even behind my back.

One morning around mid-month, I heard a deep sniff behind me. Immediately, Heather said: "Give me kids! Quit thinking about

9/11 and lend me your dick!"

I spun around and glared; a mature woman dressed in a sweater and jeans stood behind me, waiting to get some sugar for her coffee. I must have looked like murder, because she gave a nervous glance and stepped away from me. I had a very powerful urge to belt her upside the head, and I had to turn back to stirring half and half into my coffee. My entire body filled with rage. I had to go after these fucking sniffers. It wasn't enough to walk away.

For long seconds I was confused and frustrated. *Beat her ass, and the cops will come. They'll put me in jail. Heather will get me busted. They'll take everything. This is what they WANT to happen; for me to destroy myself. Then they can say, 'well, it's just that looney guy; he did it to himself.'*

Instead of attacking the woman, I made an ugly face at her. Then I sat down at a table to read a book. It was worth noting that the book was titled *Divine Fury: A History of Genius*, by Darrin M. McMahon. This was nonfiction, and the author presented ideas about geniuses from ancient times until today. The ancient Greeks and Romans thought geniuses were inspired by the gods, early Christians felt that God inspired genius, and so forth, working up to the modern day and the notion that almost everyone had the potential to be a genius in some area, if only society would invest in their education.

Reading *anything* was a difficult task, due to my illness, and that made each book more precious. As I read, my symptoms kicked up, and the voices whispered their games. My eyes roamed around the pages, trying to follow the flow of the information, but often I had to read the same paragraphs and same pages several times. Even once I read it, the information jumped around in my head. I could remember only a little of what had been written.

This said, *Divine Fury* fascinated me, and I fought my symptoms and read the pages. I hadn't known any geniuses, but might I be one? The thought was too fantastical to give any real credence to, but maybe…know what I mean? You can't just walk around claiming to be a genius; you have to prove it. Einstein wrote not one famous paper, but four! The field of physics still relies on math he did a century ago, and even though he has been dead for decades, he had a huge impact on the field.

And there's Michelangelo, and on and on. Standout talents who were head and shoulders above their peers. I read the book, wondering if I, too, could be a genius, but where was the proof? I was definitely no math genius; I could hardly balance a checkbook. I crapped out in basic algebra. But, was I a creative genius? Where was the proof?

In the meantime, the regular symptoms drove on with a fierce vengeance. When I lay down to sleep, I found no peace; instead, Heather badgered me: "THREE KIDS! Give me three goddamned kids! Redheaded babies! Why aren't you looking for your billion dollars? You'll never find it if you don't look! What do you think is going to happen, I'm just going to *give* it to you?"

Fuck off, I snapped, in my mind. *I'm in my fifties. It's too late for kids.*

"The WHOLE WORLD respects you, even when you're an asshole and don't believe me!" she hollered. "NO ONE has done as much for the human race as you! God damn it, *quit whining.*"

The voices went on and on and on, day and night. For a short few days the noise had decreased to an hour or two a day, then it came roaring back. Why? What was the trigger? Was this a natural cycle for my illness? Was talking about my illness with my friends only making it stronger?

I didn't know. But I knew I hated my illness, hated these voices and delusions. I fought them every day, and I almost always lost.

Around this time I made the decision to give up my volunteer position at the public library. No way I could pay attention to the patrons, with all the nonsense in my head. So I wrote an email to the woman who ran the gallery, and I let the position go. This meant that I had fewer reality checks on my rampaging thoughts, and I am sure this contributed to what happened next.

A few days later I starting thinking about my three years in the army, when I was an infantry soldier. This was many years ago, in my early twenties, when I held the rank of Specialist Four. Suddenly I "remembered" a conversation with the first lieutenant in charge of the platoon I served in. He had called for me to come talk, and I reported to his office. He was six or eight older than me.

Me: "Good morning, sir."

1 Lt: "Good morning, Specialist Doering. I've been thinking about some of the things you were saying during our last field problem." (A field problem is when the soldiers go out into the woods and shoot blanks at each other; it's a pretend war designed for training purposes.)

Me: "Did I say something inappropriate, sir?"

1 Lt: "Not inappropriate. Just unusual. I want you to take a test. Not with me, but with an appropriate expert. The military will pay for it."

Me: "Physical fitness test, sir?" I was fit as a fiddle and ready to show off a little bit.

1 Lt: "Mental aptitude test, Specialist. I have scheduled you for a week from today. I'll talk with your platoon sergeant and get you released from normal duties. The test will take a few hours."

Me: "Yes, sir." I looked at the ground and felt my face growing red. "Like a test for mental deficiency?" Sometimes I opened my mouth, and stupid comments came out. Had the lieutenant noticed?

1 Lt: "No, I'm looking to see if you're unusually intelligent. This test will check your math skills, verbal skills, writing skills, creativity, and so forth. I took this test once, and the results said I was above average intelligence but not a genius. Report back to me at 9a.m. sharp, next Tuesday."

Me: "Yes, sir."

To make a long story short, I took the test, and the results said I was near-genius. The major who administered the test said, "You're so close to genius that the fault could be you're not familiar with this kind of test. That probably cost you a few wrong answers. You would be well served to take it again in a couple months."

"I see, ma'am," I said. But I never took the test again.

So I "remembered" all this, in little dribs and drabs, as I slowly worked my way through *Divine Fury*. Sometimes I knew this "memory" was a delusion, but most of the time I thought it was real.

Things became even more confused. I wrote emails to my friends, describing all these symptoms, and pleading for advice. My friends said to talk to my psychiatrist and not them.

"These are just delusions," said my friend Jackie, who is bipolar herself. "Don't let them sucker you. You're stronger than them."

But I wasn't stronger; even the encouraging words couldn't throw the balance in my favor. After half a dozen more emails, I had to admit defeat. No exercises I did, no pills I took, no CBSST mental gymnastics, did more than slightly reduce the problems. Instead of further adjusting my meds and calling on friends who were showing signs of compassion fatigue, I adjusted my attitude and decided I was just going to have to live with the illness at its current intensity.

The minor voices wove their noise in and out of Heather's frequent demands. I will spare you the repetitious nature of much of what they said and pick it up when a minor voice said:

"You don't believe us, because you're missing key memories. It's like 'elimination,' but the memories stay gone for ten years."

That doesn't even make sense, I thought. *What memories?*

"The memories of when you signed on for all this. The meetings with media giants, and the president of the United States."

That isn't real, I said feebly. But it was real. I was a billionaire, and I was published in 70 languages, and people owed me. Big-time.

"We worked it all out, you and all these leaders. 'Elimination' is just a weakling version of the game that launched it all. There are some very smart psychiatrists in charge of your mental health. Billions of people know you. Everyone wants you to finish and get your goodies. No one has ever had so many supporters, ever!"

I said nothing. My friend Jackie's comment about these thoughts 'just' being delusions crossed my mind, but I had never heard of anything like what was happening to me. I had heard of cases where people thought they were Jesus, or a Rockefeller, or the president of the United States, but delusions that went on for years and years and kept building on themselves? How 'real' was this going to get, and where did it all end?

My computer kept humming as I went online and looked up my name in a search engine. The usual pages came up. Nothing about a Nobel Peace Prize, nothing about what the voices were talking about. Not a school or library or government building named after me; nothing supported the voices.

There was a side effect of talking with my friends, though: I started having intense and lengthy flashbacks to my high school days. Most of these were times I screwed up in class, or gave the wrong answer to a question from the teacher, or fell asleep in the early morning classes. The feeling of screwing up was acute and painful. Often I would have these flashbacks when I was around other people, especially at the café, so I would suddenly blurt out, "Shit. Not Heather again," and then turn red in the face. Patrons at the cafe noticed and gave me a puzzled look, and I experienced these old memories back at the same time as seeing the person in the here and now. Different times in my life superimposed on each other, so that now I got a fractured wrist in high school gym class, and at the same time I almost lost my M-16 out the side door of a helicopter in the Army, and so on. If there was purpose to these flashbacks, their logic was beyond me.

The minor voices went back to the countdown timer, and now it was like, "783, 69, 621, 66…" Was there an end date to all this? And was it really going to be months before I found out?

"It's not just *any* end-point," said a minor voice. I couldn't tell them apart. It would really be hell if all the minor voices took on more personality, so that I was fighting off a dozen of them a day.

What happens at 0? I queried them.

"You meet Heather, silly," said the voice. And the countdowns continued every day, sometimes for an hour or two and sometimes from when I woke up until I went to bed again.

Maybe it was thinking about Jesus that started the next blurry period, but I "remembered" this gem, which took place at my first job out of the army. I was a plastic craftsman who made arch supports (orthotics) for people's feet. I enjoyed this job: it was creative, took some skill so it was not boring, and the three of us who worked there (one boss, two employees) often talked as we worked. The usual topics were women, work, and random thoughts about life. So one day I said:

"I had a dream the other night."

My boss and the other employee looked at each other, because my dreams were usually weird and got a real discussion going.

Boss: "What was it?"

Other employee (OE): "Let me guess, you're gay."

Me: "I dreamed I could talk to animals."

OE: "You were an elf?"

Boss: "You must have been stoned."

Me: "I was a saint. I told a friend of mine about this, and she didn't think it was interesting. She kind of freaked out."

Boss: "This was in the dream? Or in the real world? Can you even tell the difference?"

We all laughed, and I said, "Well, I guess I daydream sometimes, but maybe I really am a saint? I should try speaking to animals and see if it works."

Boss (sternly): "You'd better lay off that talk. You go around claiming to be a saint, you'll end up locked in the bug house. Think about it. If you really were a saint, you'd feel a strong urge to become some kind of Christian. Agnostics can't be saints."

I thought it over and tried to figure out if he was right, but I eventually gave it up because I had never heard of a secular saint before. He was right, I'd have to become a Christian before I would be accepted as a saint.

So much for that.

Had this conversation ever taken place in the real world? Was this a sample of how my personality worked, years before I became mentally ill? Or was it something I dreamed up one day, under influence of the voices and the pressure they put on me to believe their stories? I still don't know, even now. And the longer this bad cycle went on, the more difficult it became to tell reality from illness.

Thanksgiving arrived, and I stood in line at Golden Hall with the homeless and the poor and the recent immigrants. There were plenty of sickly people, on crutches and in wheel chairs, and I am sure I was not the only mentally ill person waiting for dinner. The line moved at a reasonable pace, and the Salvation Army volunteers led me to a seat at a long table. It seemed that several of the grey-haired men seated across from me were veterans, and they talked about some of their experiences in the Marines and the Navy. Their conversations made the voices in my head bellow about my experiences in the Army, and I said few words to these old-timers.

Eventually a volunteer brought a plate of turkey and mashed potatoes with gravy, and green beans, and so on. I ate heartily. Most of the time I could not tell exactly where I was: back in the Army again? At a Thanksgiving dinner with my grandparents when I was a child? At Golden Hall? And who were all these people, anyway? Clearly not family, nor colleagues. Why were the volunteers all teen-agers? There were a few adults, running the show, and the rest were young people, helping out.

That got me musing on the nature of service: service in the armed forces, religious service bringing food to the poor, service as in volunteering at the library, and so on. But the thoughts ran around, and the voices barked, and I couldn't follow the ideas in any coherent manner. The only thing I was sure of was that those Christians who spent their Thanksgiving day volunteering to help out the poor and ill must have a special place in heaven.

Finally I finished eating, and I went home.

I want to finish off the miserable month of November with something I saw on the street. This took place during my morning walk. On the street near my apartment building I saw an orange tabby cat scooch along, out of the corner of my eye. I turned my head to see it better, but when I looked fully, the cat wasn't there. It was just another visual hallucination and another reminder that I was dangerously close to simply drifting away.

December: merry fucking Christmas

I prayed for a Christmas free of voices and pain, but in my heart I feared that everything was going to go sour. How long were these symptoms going to go on with such ferocity, like a swarm of stinging wasps? Surely the voices were wearing themselves out? Wasn't Heather due to give me a break?

Instead, things went sideways. Sitting one morning at the café, I overheard someone talking about earning a Ph.D. This made me think of a friend of mine who looked into doing a Ph.D. in engineering, and I was struck by the "realization" that I wanted to do a Ph.D. too. Just like that, out of nowhere.

Later that day I looked up Ph.D. programs in anthropology, because my masters degree is in anthropology, and it seemed like good sense to build on that. In particular I had studied socio-cultural anthropology, which is comprised of projects like going to the Maya Indians of Central America and recording their stories and songs.

Earning a Ph.D. was a daunting prospect. I have been interested in the Maya Indians since I was a teenager, and I've read a lot of books and magazine articles on these people, but to go pro was a serious step. Before I got in over my head, it seemed like a good idea to explore where I wanted to get my doctorate.

An hour later I had finished my morning walk and was at home again, sitting in front of my computer. I plugged some terms into a search engine, and it didn't take long to single out a few universities. Two were state schools, and one was an Ivy: namely, Harvard. Then I went to the web sites of these universities and looked at their anthropology programs and how much it would cost to earn a doctorate. As you'd expect, Harvard was the most expensive, by far. For some reason, that made it more attractive.

Armed with this knowledge, I shot off emails to friends, discussing this new fascination. They asked me, had I already applied? When was the application deadline?

Back to the web sites, only to find out that the application deadline for the 2016 fall semester had already passed. So it was pointless worrying about it for seven or eight months.

Could I really get into Harvard?

Heather came to visit, in my mind: "Have you considered that 9/11 might not have ever happened?" she said nonchalantly. "I wouldn't talk about it with other people, if I were you. That's a good way to end up in the looney bin. Just think about fake news events, all day, all night." This was in the café, in the early afternoon. I was reading some print-outs from Harvard's web site and dreaming of going Ivy.

I've been there, I thought back at her. *I've been to the reflecting pools.*

"Are you sure?" she said. "Sometimes a break with reality can seem pretty realistic."

It's you who are not real, I said. This fixation on doing a Ph.D. had given me some courage. I had done well in my masters program, and I felt I could do well in a doctoral program.

"GIVE ME KIDS!" she yelped. Her auburn hair went frizzy and wild, and she looked like a madwoman.

GIVE ME MY BILLION DOLLARS! I yelled back at her.

"THREE KIDS! OR NO NOBEL PRIZE!"

Now, I wanted that Nobel. I wanted it *bad.* Hadn't I done enough to earn it? The whole world had changed, due to me, and the bastards had hidden my memories and were holding my prizes and awards and cash.

Give me my fucking prize, I snarled.

"Come to L.A. and fuck me," she teased. "We can talk about short stories."

She went on in this vein, hour after hour, day after day. I listened to her sometimes and managed to block her off or drive her away with CBSST techniques sometimes. But she was LOUD, and persistent, and came back almost every day. Thus the first week of

December passed.

One of my old friends from college lived a few miles up the highway from my place, and he had a daughter who was six years old. She was deeply into an animated kids' movie called *Brave*, which features a girl who is keen on bow and arrows. So my goddaughter wanted a bow for Christmas. I ordered one for her, and it came in the mail, and I wrapped it in Christmas paper and set it aside.

"Yes," my friend said on the phone, as we discussed the upcoming holiday. "We're staying in town this year, and you're invited to Christmas dinner. I don't know the details yet. Did you get my daughter a bow? You used common sense and got her those arrows that end in a suction cup, right? Not a sharp tip?"

"Of course," I said.

"Still hearing voices? Still bad?"

"It's pretty wretched," I said, not really wanting to go into detail. I noticed that when I talked about the symptoms at length, that tended to trigger the voices to come and wreak havoc in my mind.

"I'll call you before the holiday and let you know what time to show up," he said, and he broke the connection.

The weather seemed quite cold for San Diego, and things went sideways again. I realized I didn't *need* a Ph.D. Since I was worth a billion dollars, I could fund my own archaeological expeditions into the jungles of Central America. We could bring back tons of jade and painted pottery and carved stone statues. Money opens many closed doors, and my expeditions would rival the National Geographic Society's digs.

But a Ph.D. would show I was one of the best-educated people in America. Earning the degree would be a pride point, and it would reflect well on my family. So far as I knew, there wasn't a single doctorate in the entire extended family. I would have bragging rights for the rest of my life. I was interested in making a contribution to the field of anthropology, and take a chance to study the Maya Indians more deeply, but I wasn't a madman when I did my masters degree.

That is to say, I'm mentally ill, not stupid, and although I have frequent delusions, I am not completely cut off from reality. After a week of exploring a Ph.D. in anthropology, it occurred to me to wonder how the hell I was going to undertake a doctorate degree, with all that work, when my head was terribly screwed up? Every day voices hijacked my mind, I experienced constant paranoia, and on and on. And even if I received financial aid, that only covered tuition and school expenses. It didn't cover living expenses. The more I thought about what was involved in getting the Ph.D., the more it seemed, well, *nuts.*

About this time, when my fantasies of getting a doctorate were flagging, I saw an article online. It was about mentally ill people and the police. The title was: "People with mental illness 16 times more likely to be killed by police." According to the article, if you were mentally ill and had any kind of encounter with the police, the cops were 16 times more likely to shoot you dead than if you were a mentally healthy citizen. The cops said there are two important factors that leads to our being killed: we do weird and sometimes hostile things, and we don't obey commands from the police.

There were some numbers to quantify the carnage: about one in four people killed by the police was mentally ill. In 2015, the police killed about 1,000 people in the United States. So some 250 mentally ill people died in the hands of the police. And this goes on *every year.*

I read this article. I re-read it. This was the first time I had thought about such issues, and I wondered if I was a good target for a police killing. Sometimes I talked to myself, or talked to Heather or the other voices as I walked to the grocery store and back, or on my daily walk. If I was deep in the grip of paranoia, how would I respond to a couple of cops drawing their guns and shouting out commands?

It was clear that I had to be very wary of the police. They were literally gunning for people like me.

A few days later I completed editing the novel I had been working on all year, and I sent it through the production process with CreateSpace, which is a self-publishing venture set up by Amazon. With all the mental illness I had been experiencing, I had barely been able to keep up work on the novel, but I had finished it after all. I ordered a proof print, and it arrived in the mail and looked good. It took only a few minutes of my time to approve the book and make it available to readers on Amazon. I told my friends and family that it was for sale, and they ordered some copies. So I managed some tenuous connection with reality in spite of all the mental illness.

The loose paranoia I felt about the cops gave way to more specific paranoia about the media. Around the 20th of the month I sat down in the café at five in the morning to read a book about geniuses, and someone sniffed, right behind me.

"We owe you," said a flat voice that sounded nearby, though only the sniffer was close to me. Or was it, "We own you?"

"You'll get your money, someday," said a different voice.

"Heaven," said a third voice. As in, 'it's heaven with Heather.'

I started getting annoyed with these attacks.

The person behind me sniffed again, and I knew he was sucking up my thoughts to report to media people.

"They do it all for you," said the sniffer.

I turned around to see a white-haired, rough-looking fellow who was poorly dressed for the chill. It struck me that he was probably homeless, spending what little money he had for a cup of coffee and the chance to get in out of the cold.

"G'morning," he said, and then he finished getting condiments for his coffee and shuffled away to sit at a table. Did he then say, "It's your media," or was that me mumbling to myself?

All the pieces fell into place. The people who were talking were inserting thoughts into my head, and the sniffers sucked up my reactions to those thoughts. These were sorted through by psychologists, who forwarded them to famous writers, rich actors, and wild musicians to be turned into books, movies, and songs that were targeted just to me. So they did it all for me, but they did it by *torturing* me first, by invading my privacy and forcing themselves into my mind, over and over again.

I thought maybe I should throw my cup of hot coffee in the homeless guy's face. I felt resentment, and a lot of anger, at these people. Heather said I had "signed on" for this abuse and didn't remember it, but that seemed like a poor excuse for such suffering. She and her minor voices were summoned by these people, and they went after me *every day* for hours a day. What the hell was I supposed to do? If I attacked them, the cops would lock me up: I'd lose what little freedom I still had. And I was 16 times more likely to be killed by the cops in the first place.

It looked like all of society was going after me, like it or not, and all I could do was grit and grin or be killed.

My friend Daniel called. "Come to our place around five," he said. "Does the bus run on Christmas day?"

"Yes," I said. "I think it's hourly service. I might not be there right around five, but within an hour either way."

"See you then," he said.

A few days before Christmas I went to a nice restaurant for dinner. Heather didn't show up, but the minor voices went on and on: "small dinner"

"why didn't you order fish?"

"didn't you have scallops last year?"

"this place is expensive"

"where is Heather?"

"your dad is really sick, and here you sit eating good food" "loser"

"why do you still walk every day? you're not losing weight"

"did you take your pills today? bet you didn't"

"it's been months since you've seen your goddaughter—bet she doesn't even recognize you anymore"

I cut up the large sea-scallops and ate them and enjoyed every bit of the meal, in spite of the voices. It seemed strange that Heather wasn't sounding off, but of course I didn't know what she was planning for the future, either. Could hallucinations make plans? This notion seemed absurd, but I wouldn't put it past her.

Christmas day came around, and I took the bow and arrow set and rode public transportation to my friend's condo. He and his wife welcomed me, and I gave the wrapped gift to my goddaughter, who shook it and asked,

"What is it?"

"You have to wait until later to find out," said my friend, and he put it under the Christmas tree with a large number of other gifts.

"One of these days soon, the gypsies are coming for your goddaughter," said Heather in a vicious tone. She stood just off to the side of my friends, wearing cut-off shorts and sandals and a frilly blouse. She had her arms crossed in front of her chest.

Her words alarmed me, and I thought back at her, *Fuck you.*

"Come to L.A., and I'll protect her," she said.

My goddaughter looked at me expectantly, and I realized she had said something.

"What was that?" I asked her.

"Did anyone get *you* a present?" she asked.

"My parents gave me a present, and some of my friends gave me cards," I said to her.

She ran off and got a grab bag full of goodies, with Belgian chocolate as the highlight. This she presented to me, and I thanked her.

"Don't say 'thanks,' Heather hissed. "Say 'good-bye.'"

Stay out of my fucking head, I thought.

"Dinner is ready," said my friend's wife, and she set the ham and the tofurky and some veggies on the table.

My friends and I talked, and I said to my goddaughter, "I hope you get everything you want."

She smiled and said, "Grandpa got me a gift, too."

"I'm thinking, a shoot-out between organized crime and the cops, and all the stray bullets hit this condo," Heather snapped. "They're coming for you, guy, and I own all of them."

"three wise men" said a minor voice

"are you a wise man? i think you're a fool"

"omnicide"

"You've known these people a long time, but what have they ever done for you?" This was Heather, in an ugly tone of voice.

At that point I fell out of the conversation with my friends, and the voices owned me. Heather's comment bit deep and drew me into that view. It seemed everyone had failed me. The shrinks at the VA hadn't cured my illness in 9 years of trying, and my friends couldn't really say much more than, "Talk with your shrink." I felt it was my responsibility to take care of myself.

All of a sudden I thought that my illness was like having a broken leg, and every day I had to hobble to the pharmacy to get my medicine to cure my broken leg. It was *possible* to do this, but painful and time-consuming. I spent a large part of my day dealing with symptoms and trying to live a lifestyle that supported healing.

Heather's tone became cheerful. "You should commit suicide," she suggested. "Why go on with this shit? Illness, pain, feeling bad every day, people don't understand you…and the cops go out of their way to kill guys like you."

I'm going to win, I thought back at her. *I'm not always going to be ill.*

"You poor stupid dipshit," she hissed, and her voice sank into my mind like a combat knife sinks through flesh. "You have nothing.

Half-assed friends, half-assed VA, half-assed family… Like you said, you have a broken leg, and all they do is stick a Band-Aid on it. You need *strong* medicine. You need all Heather's love. I can do it for you. I can heal you completely. Shit, how many meds have you been through? Half a dozen? At least. You're willing to try new drugs. Now try me. Don't force me to hurt your friends."

I sat there for the next hour, as my friend told some funny stories about his job, and his wife, who is Japanese-American, told us about the seaweed she had cooked up as a side dish. My goddaughter wanted to open presents and kept eyeing up the pile of gifts.

And I missed almost all of it, due to the voices carrying on.

"Let's sing a little song from my childhood," Heather said, and then she didn't wait for an answer but sang some ditty that I didn't recognize. "I have a sister," she said, but that only confused me, because I didn't remember her saying that before.

"Every time you fight me, you get a little sicker," she said. "I take over another tiny piece of you."

The dinner went on, and I realized that I wasn't going to get a break. The good food, the conversation with friends, the glass of red wine; all of it was failing to tame my symptoms.

"Kill your goddaughter," Heather hissed. "You've got a steak knife. Cut her goddamned throat."

"Do you want to open a gift?" asked my friend, to his daughter.

"Yeah. Uncle Randal's first." So she tore the wrapper off and triumphantly took out the bow and arrow. "Now I'm brave, too," she said. She ran around for a while shooting the sucker cup arrows at the television and various pieces of furniture. She returned to the tree and set my gift down and opened the others and was hugely pleased.

Heather came closer. All of a sudden Uncle Ray was there, in my head. He was dressed as usual in jungle fatigues, and his face was covered in black and green camouflage. He held a combat knife in one hand and a grenade in the other hand. Jungle growth surrounded him.

"She's on her way," he said, and then he took off into the foliage. "I'm going to hold her off."

In the real world, my goddaughter talked about Christmas, but I could no longer hear her. The image of the jungle had captivated my mind. During my time in the Army, I had taken jungle warfare training in Panama. Something about the jungle appealed to me; it was dense growth, and there were lots of interesting animals and tropical birds. Uncle Ray had fought in that environment, and his memories were not so fond.

"Go back where you came from," Uncle Ray said to Heather, somewhere off in the jungle.

"I *belong* here," she said. "I *own* this guy."

I stayed where I was, in the jungle superimposed on my friends' dining room. My goddaughter and her parents were still talking about something or other.

"Now beat it, or I'll whoop your ass," Uncle Ray shouted.

Heather was gone from my mind, then; this was the firmest victory against her I had yet experienced.

Uncle Ray said, "You just have to take a firm tone of voice, that's all. No need for violence, when threats will do." Then he was gone. Didn't say good-bye, nothing. Just disappeared.

Heather appeared next to the dining table and said, "You know, your goddaughter isn't really very bright. She'll accept any mass-produced, cheap plastic bullshit. It's up to you to introduce her to a better caliber of gift, and you're failing at it. You're failing as a friend, too. When is the last time you said *anything* useful to your friends?"

Maybe if you got the fuck out of my head, I'd be able to—

"Oh, it's me? You don't like it when I'm here, and you spend all your time when I'm away wondering when I'll be back, and you hate my friends, and let me just tell you, you're ours. We own your brain, we give you the real information on how the world works, and one day we will send you to an afterlife where you will be respected."

"I'm going to win the Nobel Prize," I sort of half-whispered at my friend, but he was watching his daughter shoot arrows and didn't hear me. Or maybe he did hear me and didn't want to deal with my illness on Christmas day.

I knew that if I stayed, the voices would drone on and on and on for the rest of my evening.

"You know, I think that good dinner is wiping me out," I said to my friend.

"Ready to go home?" he asked.

"If you don't mind."

"Bye, Uncle Randal," my goddaughter said. "Thanks for the bow and arrows."

I hugged her, and my friend's wife, and then my friend drove me back to my apartment building. We made plans to go hiking sometime in the next month, and I got out of the car.

From there I took a shower, and then Heather laughed and laughed. "Your dinner was all fucked up, you didn't hear a word your friends said, and I spotted you a little time with your goddaughter. I decide what you get and what you don't get, and when. Merry fucking Christmas, asshole."

January 2016: crawling out of the slime

I celebrated New Year's Eve with a couple glasses of red wine and some cheese, and I watched the ball drop in New York City. There were no voices, not even Heather, but I did not expect this reprieve to last very long. My symptoms just didn't work that way. In my mind, it was time for this down cycle to come to an end, but I had only been under attack for four months, and that would be a short down cycle. So I could be due for another couple months yet.

Just thinking about more bad symptoms on the way made me unhappy. Heather had seemed cheerful at Christmas, but as usual, her good mood came at my expense. So I didn't know if she was going to crank up the ugliness dial, or if some new symptom would reveal itself.

As the first few days of the new year unfolded, I started having "memories" of high school and some of my friends from back then. There was a regular group of us who played a game called Dungeons and Dragons on the weekends. Parts of the "memories" seemed authentic, like talking with my friends and playing the game. Other parts seemed like pieces from someone else's life.

In these intrusive "memories," there was another high school kid named Andy something-or-other. He wasn't really a friend; he didn't play the game with us. But in school, he was loud about how much the game sucked, and what kind of losers play Dungeons and Dragons, and so forth. On Monday mornings, before classes, he would hang out in the halls at school and seek me out. A typical session went like this:

Andy: "What kind of jerk-off queers play Dungeons and Dragon? Oh, did your *dwarf* thief butt-fuck your *elf* warrior? Are they going to be married now? Can't you live in the real world? What the *fuck* are you going to do when it comes time to get a real job?"

Me: "If you don't play the game, what do you do with your free time?"

Andy belched. His breath stank of alcohol, as it usually did on Mondays, and his eyes were bleary and bloodshot. He reached out and shoved me away from him. "Fu-fu-ck you. Faggot little game. I'm smarter at seventeen than you'll ever be, your whole life. Loser. Got your books for class? Going to American History? I'm going to *gifted* classes. I should look you up when we're forty, see how I left you in the dust."

This sort of intrusive "memory" went on for a week, with Andy becoming increasingly drunk and increasingly violent. He knocked the books out of my hands; he slapped one of my friends across the face. The incidents reeled off one after the next, day after day.

I couldn't remember with certainty what year of high school all this took place, and I felt that I was under attack by a drunken bully and a vicious mental illness at the same time. In the "memories" I fought back but always lost. Heather didn't comment on these scenes, but the minor voices pointed out all my failings as a human being. If this was a symptom, it was a symptom of what?

Then one day Andy brought a combat knife to school and said he was going to kill one of the teachers. He showed the knife to me, and I told a friend, who took the situation to a teacher. In no time the cops were at the school. One cop had Andy in handcuffs, and the other went to talk with the principal. Here's how the scene played out:

Cop: "And you say this knife was just for show? You were just joking?"

Andy: "Randal, you're next, mother fucker. You'll see that knife again, real close."

One of my friends (to the cop): "Andy says things like this all the time, officer. He threatens teachers, threatens us. One of these days he'll be so drunk he'll actually kill somebody."

Cop: "Nothing wrong with having a few drinks. Life can be harsh. I suggest you mind your own business, kid."

Teacher: "So what's the best thing for us to do, file a complaint? And what will that accomplish?"

Cop: "He didn't actually hurt anyone. You can see he's just had a few too many. I've done that, you've done that, probably every person in this school has gone on at least one bender in their life. Here's what I'll do: I'll go pick up my partner, and we'll take this guy and put him in the drunk tank until tomorrow. Phone his parents and let them decide to come get him or let him sleep it off. See what he says then. My guess is, he'll straighten up."

Teacher: "That's it? Brings a knife to school and threatens to kill people, and nothing happens? What would happen to me if I did that?"

Cop: "He'll shape up!" He gave the teacher an evil eye while Andy leered.

Andy: "No one gives a shit about teachers or students. You're all expendable. The police are morally bankrupt. I could have killed all of you, and they wouldn't have even arrested me." He looked upset, and then he threw up on the floor. The stench of far too much alcohol soaked into the air.

Cop: "See? Listen to him, he's just drunk. Let's go." He jerked the handcuffs, and Andy's face took on a miserable look. The two of them went down the hall and disappeared into the crowd of high school kids.

Teacher: "How do you like that? I guess we shouldn't bother calling the police until someone is dead. Then they'll say, why didn't you call in and report that this kid had a weapon?"

My friend: "I thought something more was required, too. Now Andy is going to feel empowered, because he'll know he can get away with it."

I was disturbed by the intensity of these "memories," and I didn't trust the way reality and paranoid delusions wove in and out of each other. Was "Andy" even a real person? Had he really come to school every day drunk, and he never got into trouble for it?

So I sent emails to friends from that period of my life, and they got back to me. Two of them said they remembered him, and they said that he was a petty criminal during his high school years, but they didn't remember him brandishing weapons or threatening to kill people.

Reality continued to warp, for me. I was still reading books about geniuses, and around mid-January I "realized" that I was a genius, too. Hadn't I taken that test in the Army? Wasn't I reading books about geniuses, and it seemed that all the descriptions were about me?

The nagging question kept coming up, *where's the proof?* I considered writing to the Department of the Army and asking for a copy of the IQ test I took, but I knew that probably would be a waste of time. The Army had forms online that you could download and fill out, to request copies of certain documents that pertained to your military service, but I felt confident that an IQ test result wouldn't be such a record. If I had taken the test to begin with...

Given my poor math grades all through school, I was not the next Einstein. But as an artist, I had something. I had proof. Long ago I wrote a book about a Maya Indian boy and his family. It's fiction, written like an auto-biography. And it's illustrated with hundreds of paintings, captions, touches of calligraphy, and so on. Taken as a whole, this unusual work had to be proof that I was a genius. Hot damn! I had to be 200 IQ or more! Not that pesky 150 bullshit. All you had to do was read the book, and you'd see it for yourself!

But I had doubts, and as a few more days went by, those doubts grew. I had shown that book to many people. I had put a version of it on my website for people to download and read, and I put a text-only version on Smashwords, where it had been downloaded more than a hundred times. People were looking at it, they were interested in it…so why weren't *they* calling me a genius? It was suspect that I was my own cheering section. I read more books about geniuses, but the certainty that I was a genius faded into the background.

I decided that this year I would only work on some short stories. No novel. Every year that I worked on a novel, it was a hard fight against mental illness to complete that work and bring it to market. With the symptoms as nasty as they had been, this fight had really worn me out. I was going to do some easy stories, and that had to be enough.

One chilly January morning at mid-month, while I was walking my usual exercise route in San Diego, I had a vivid flashback to Andy and one of his friends ambushing me in the parking lot of my old high school. This was winter, in the town of Durango, Colorado. The parking lot was plowed, but there was a lot of snow everywhere else. As I walked toward the front doors, Andy and his friend ran from behind a parked truck and slammed into me. I fell down, and they kicked and pounded and beat me. I fought back as best I could. Then the bell rang to announce ten minutes to the start of class. Andy and his accomplice took off into the building, and I picked myself up and went inside. I went to American History, and that's when I realized my nose was bleeding a great deal. All the students looked at me, and when the teacher came in, the same teacher from the other Andy "memory," he said, "I suppose that was Andy?"

"With a friend," I muttered.

"Did they have weapons? I don't know why I'm asking, the cops won't do anything until someone is dead."

"No," I said.

"You're a mess. Do you want to go to the school nurse?"

"No. I've got a Kleenex."

"Then let's get started on today's class, everyone."

For some reason, these "memories" about high school just kept going. Every day, for hours, I would relive classes, and have chats with teachers from thirty years ago, and have fights with Andy.

These situations were my dominant symptoms, but they were not all the delusions I went through. The minor voices came back around the 20th.

"you speak 5 languages" one of them said. I *knew* they were telling me the truth, but when I tried to speak Mayan, or even Spanish, all I could produce was some half-witted mumbling of a few words or phrases. And when I asked, "What are the five languages?" the minor voice seemed to make up a different list each time.

"Nobel Peace Prize," it said. And where *was* my Nobel? Away somewhere else, in the future. If it existed at all.

"knighted by the Queen" It *felt* like any day now someone from Buckingham Palace would call up to congratulate me and send me a ticket to England for the knighting ceremony.

And of course, there was a minor voice that whispered, "Presidential Medal of Freedom with distinction" But I received not one peep from the White House.

"play 5 musical instruments at ~~professional~~ *genius* level" So when I went to Amazon music online, why weren't any of my CDs for sale there?

There were always explanations from the voices: "Your new skills are *hidden*, like the memories of meeting with world leaders. They're hidden behind a mental firewall. When it's time, you'll get them back. You have a lot to look forward to!"

"Heather loves you"

The claims were so ridiculous that I had to laugh at them, but I believed in them, too. The voices were *intimate*. They seemed like old friends, and they knew me very well. They could sound off day or night, when I was at my best and at my worst, and they could always excuse their own excesses by blaming them on Heather.

My delusions continued, in episodes that went on in short segments each day. It was still winter in Durango, and Andy decided to up the ante. This was on another Monday morning, and everyone put their coats and boots away and got their books. Andy staggered up to me and tried to knock the books out of my hands, but he was so drunk that he just sort of fumbled and hit his head on my locker door. As usual, he looked like he'd been on a weekend bender.

"Fu-fu-ck you!" he screeched in a blast of alcoholic breath. "Cops on my side!" He took a swing at me and hit me dead-on in the solar plexus, and the air went out of me. Other students stopped what they were doing and looked to see what was happening.

Andy punched me in the head a few times and grabbed hold of me and tried to knock me down.

The air came back into my lungs, and I shoved him away from me. "Andy, this has to stop," I said. "Just go to class."

"I'm in the *gifted* classes," he burbled. "I'm *better* than you."

"Go to class," I repeated, and I started to walk away.

He punched me in the back, and for some reason that blow finally made me mad. I dropped my books and turned around and punched him in the face. He was so blotto that he could hardly stand up to start with, and I had the guilty feeling that I was taking advantage of a drunk, but I started pounding on him. Blows to the face, jabs to the ribs, crack to the nose.

His eyes widened, and he tried to speak but only drooled. I punched him in the mouth, and I said, "*Fuck off*, Andy." Then I shoved him with both hands, and he fell over onto his butt. The fight was over. He passed out, and that was that. I picked up my books and went to class, and Andy did not trouble me anymore. Like many bullies, he just had to see me stand up for myself.

Could geniuses really have false memories? Where did memories end and delusions begin? The high school was real. My friends were real. So why "remember" some bully who half my friends said didn't act as I remembered him acting? Was this really about Heather and her minor voices rolling through my mind, filling my head with junk whenever they wished?

Those delusions went on for weeks, day after day. They played, and played again with minor changes, then new versions began. I had no idea why I thought of high school, or Andy, to begin with. That had been a long time ago, and nothing useful had come of it.

Literary genius. Delusion, or fact? I opened the electronic files of the book I had written that I felt might be a work of genius, and I looked at the layouts and the sumptuous pictures I had created. I had sent this book out to literary agents, a few years ago, and the few who responded told me that it didn't fit the acceptable categories for the industry. One agent said the graphics were attractive, but it was more an art book than something that could be mass marketed. So, no, she would not represent this work to publishers.

Somewhere in my gut, I was sure my book was outstanding and powerful. But didn't every author feel this way about their work? Hell, every artist working in every medium thought they were a genius! But in reality, only the rare individual was proclaimed to be that bright, and certainly no one was running around screaming, "Randal Doering! A genius for our times!" It would be nice if that happened, but I wasn't holding my breath.

Near the end of January, at the café, Uncle Ray appeared in my mind, standing in the jungle. His fatigues were disheveled, and he hadn't shaved in a while. He carried a combat knife and wore brand-new jungle boots. The look on his face could have killed a man. He had a terrible intensity to him that said he was planning murder.

"She's coming, and this time I'm going after her with stealth," he whispered to me.

"Three kids, goddamn it!" Heather howled. She was in the distance, in the lush jungle growth, and Uncle Ray put one finger to his lips in a "shush" sign and then loped off into the foliage.

There was a single loud gunshot, and a minute later Heather danced into the small clearing in front of me. She had a bloody scratch on her face, I assumed from Uncle Ray. She wore a tight sun-yellow dress that showed off her curves very nicely, and she looked like she always did, young and pretty and unperturbed.

"Guess how much you're worth?" she asked me.

I accepted that Uncle Ray was dead or taken out, and it would be a while before I saw him again. If ever. *I'm not worth much of anything,* I thought.

"Three billion dollars," she said. "Hollywood is making whole movies about your Uncle Ray, and you get a cut. It's their way of thanking a generation for the sacrifices they made in Vietnam."

I'm a genius, I thought at her.

She made a sour face and shook her head. Then I returned to sipping my coffee, and she left.

As January closed, my symptoms became less severe and less frequent. The voices went back to their oldest games, saying bad things about everyone or mocking what I said. This return to basics depressed me. It was like starting a bad cycle all over again, or crawling out of the slime twice. I wanted peace in my own mind, but I was sure I wasn't going to get it.

February: someday things will be better

February started off on a positive note, with a reduction in the intensity of symptoms. But I knew that could change in an instant, and I had ongoing paranoia involving the anniversary of my illness.

The 7th of February came along, and I paused in my life to note that I had been ill ten years, with schizoaffective disorder. Ten years ago that day I had awakened in the early hours of the morning and spent the next several hours listening to a voice in my mind. Things had degenerated from there.

I felt like I deserved some sort of award for surviving this whole time. Years of unemployment, homelessness, loss of all my money, constant hallucinations, voices, paranoia, and delusions, extreme poverty, friends abandoning me or telling me go somewhere else, living in a culvert…the nightmare seemed endless, and I felt that some recognition was due, even if the only person who cared was me. So in a way, February 7th was a triumph: I had survived.

That feeling of victory fell apart, though, when I asked what were the next ten years going to be like? When I talked to my friends about my fears for the future—return to homelessness, full break with reality, manic spending sprees, cops shooting me, and on and on—my friends said to do the best I could, and deal with the bad stuff as it arose. Don't go courting trouble.

I needed a touch of humor in my life, and accordingly I picked up a copy of a book called *Everything I Need to Know I Learned From Dungeons and Dragon,* by Shelly Mazzanoble. It is a funny take on your basic mainstream American young woman looking for love and dealing with her difficult mother, and playing Dungeons and Dragons. The book started out slow, but it became funnier as it went, and soon it did something amazing: it broke through the pains my illness inflicted on me and made me laugh.

After a week of lightweight symptoms, I dreamed about a more amusing session of Dungeons and Dragons. This was in my teen years in Colorado, when half a dozen of us played the game at the Durango Public Library every Sunday. There were five guys (including me) and two gals playing the game, when we stopped for a break. It went like this:

Sean said, "Randal, you suck as the dungeon master. You have all these weird interpretations of the rules. We should elect someone king, and that person should decide whenever there's a quibble."

Dorothea burst out laughing and said, "Yeah, king of the nerds."

And I said, "Yeah, that's me. I'm king of the nerds."

Stace immediately said, "I'll vote for Randal."

Sean abstained. "Let's not vote for *such* a nerd for king of the nerds."

Jay said, "That works for me."

Angel laughed and said, "It would never work if one of us *girls* was king."

Angel said, "It's either Jay or Randal. Sean, are you sure you're not voting? We could throw this!"

Sean snickered. "No way."

Dorothea said, "Well, I vote for Randal."

Chuck threw down his pen and said, "Why does he get to be king of the nerds? I wanted it."

Dorothea said, "Because he grabbed it first."

"So what does that leave me?" Chuck said.

"What should we call you, Chuck?" said Michael. "Toady, or lackey? Or lack-wit, that's even better."

"I'll be king of the nerds," Chuck said.

"You got not one vote," Stace pointed out.

"Phooey, I don't need votes. I'm king. It's a coup. Suck it up, Randal."

"Since you're not choosing, I say you're a toady," said Sean. "The king's toady."

"Phooey on you, Sean. King! I'm king, everybody."

"Quick, Chuck, what sound do toadies make?" said Sean.

"Randal's quicker than you, Chuck," said Dorothea.

"Ouch!" Chuck said. "Quicker, how?"

"In the game. He thinks his way around the monsters really fast. Anyone else with me?" asked Dorothea.

"Randal's quicker," said Stace. "Not by a lot, but by enough to count."

"Randal's way faster," said Sean. "What say you, toady?"

"I hate to say it, but Randal got there quicker than you, Chuck," said Jay. "Are you saying you didn't notice this?"

At this point Chuck became annoyed. "Sean got all of you stirred up. That's all. He's instigating."

"That's me," said Sean with a grin. "What was that, toady?"

"You're all against me?" Chuck said. "Why?"

"You make a better toady than Randal would," said Dorothea.

Chuck looked frustrated. "Well, damn. Burned by the girls, no less. I guess I say, 'rebbit.'"

This "memory" didn't come back all in one dream. It returned in pieces, one night's incidents blurring into the next night's dialogue fading into a focus on each individual and what they said.

I was amazed at the humor of this episode, because 90% of what happened in my schizoaffective mind was negative and ugly. It was like there was a filter in my brain that kept humor out or turned it into something loathsome. This incident about the king of the nerds made me laugh. After this dream had gone on a few nights, I sent emails to some of my old friends, asking them if they remembered this incident. No one did.

I wondered why I had these "returning memories," what purpose they served my ailing brain. Did this touch of humor mean the worst of this down cycle was over? Was Heather going to be funny from now on? Was the illness going to break down for good? I actually became excited by these thoughts, because times had been bad for so long. I read Shelley's book, and I got humor. Maybe I needed to learn from this, and change my whole life?

Alas, the illness was not going to let this happen. I finished Shelley's book and gave it to the library, to pass on the laughs to others, and then I thought, *I haven't learned half of what there is to know about geniuses. Let's take a look.* So I sat down on a library computer and typed in some search phrases, and that was how I ended up with a couple more books on genius. And that was how the illness hijacked what looked like an easy road to better days. It wasn't that I was back to thinking of myself as a genius; it was more like a sudden interest in a subject I had not thought about much before.

With my interest in high IQ's came thoughts of how much money your average genius must make as they patented their inventions, wrote their bestsellers, and published their mathematical flights of fancy. I wondered how much house I could buy with my billion dollars. I wasn't interested in *big*; I was interested in *quality*. I found some articles on the web that showed a few of the most spectacular private libraries in the world, and the photos were breathtaking. Gorgeous woodwork, amazing doors of metal or wood, globes of the Earth and of Mars, and of course, bookcases filled with cherished volumes.

I scoffed at rich people spending $90 million on a 300-room mansion or on a fleet of 50 antique cars, and I looked at pictures of some of these overblown palaces just to see how these people wasted their money. Of course, to many people a private library looked like a waste of time, too.

The voices were still around, but they had quieted down. The minor voices came to play games, drilling their buzz words into my mind and setting off painful thoughts of burning book cases and mansions attacked by armies of thieves.

As the month reached the halfway point, Heather showed up. She had dressed in a sun-yellow miniskirt and had white socks and black shoes. Her blouse was a shade of light purple and was cut low in front.

"Not so stupid anymore, eh? Now you're looking for ways to spend your cash. A billion dollars will go a *long* way, won't it?"

"I feel better," I blurted. This was in my room, in front of my computer.

"Of course you feel better, you're going along with us. You can fight us and make yourself more sick, or you can do what we want, and we'll support you." She smiled, but it was not friendly; it was just a phony leer.

I continued to look at houses of the wealthy. There were tons of articles about this subject on the internet, and many of them had very engaging images to go with the words. Inlaid floors in dark or light wood, spacious writing desks, and statues of marble, granite, or even mahogany. I greedily consumed these sites, day after day, as I planned to buy some old Victorian house somewhere and turn it into an architectural masterpiece.

Heather showed up sometimes and commented on what I was doing, like this: "Why do you keep focusing on libraries? I mean, fuck, I'm a journalist, and I enjoy books, but if it was *me* looking for a house, I'd check out the kitchen and living room. Can you say HDTV?"

"If I had a good library, I'd probably live in it," I said. I meant this to be funny, but she didn't even chuckle.

"You know, for someone who is well read, and has a masters degree, you're kind of stupid," she said on another day. "You read the newspaper, right? You see that cops have turned into the biggest thieves of all. Police seize *billions* of dollars in assets every year, and most of the people they grab from are innocent. The cops just take everything they can get, and if you try to stop them, they gun you down. What do you think of that?"

"Where did you hear that?" I asked. "What do you expect me to say? What anyone would say: there should be limits on what the cops can seize. Due process, or something. I'm not a legal expert."

"No, just a pansy little reader who wants to bury his face in fantasy all day and pretend we can all ignore the real world."

Through an ongoing haze of comments like this one, I read the books on geniuses, and I guess I was learning something, because the voices began incorporating the most interesting facts into their daily harassment:

"women geniuses," one voice jabbed at me. That is, according to one expert, only about 3% of geniuses were female. This struck me as so biased and misogynist that I could hardly hear this without getting really hacked off.

"30%, 70%," said another voice. That is, scientists now consider genius to be about one third genetics and two-thirds environmental factors. This made me flash back to my dad buying me books on ancient civilization like Egypt and the Maya Indians, when I was growing up. He fed my interests, and thus my family environment was supportive. Many people are not so fortunate.

"poor, mad poets," purred a third voice. I felt pretty sure this one was Heather in disguise. In one study of poets, 87% suffered severe mental illness at some point in their lives.

"I'm not going to run around feeling sorry for myself," I snarled under my breath. "Creative people have it hard, but so does everyone else. No one here gets out alive."

Heather laughed and laughed. "You're the one thinks he's a genius. You dumb fucking ass wipe. You're nothing but a lunatic, half a step from raving homelessness. You're *our* lunatic, until we let you go. Some day we will let you into the system, but *guess what?* That day isn't today and it probably isn't even this year."

Then she took off, and I went back to reading.

As I lived through the last week of February, I noticed that the voices didn't attack as vigorously or as often as they had just a few weeks before hand. I didn't dare hope that I was at an end to this down cycle, but I thought maybe I had a reprieve—a week or two— when the symptoms wouldn't hound me to exhaustion every day.

"Someday things will get better," Heather smirked, somewhere out of sight, in some dark corner of my mind.

One last tidbit from the books on geniuses: geniuses are much more prone to mental illness than the general population. The exact percentages vary wildly, depending on what kind of geniuses are being examined, but if you are a genius, odds are you will suffer mental illness sometime in your life.

The fact that I spent more time each day in conversation with voices in my head than dealing with the real world and the people in it, confirmed for me that I must be a genius.

March: a cure is near?

San Diego has moderate weather year-round, and I like it that way. If I want to experience snow I go up into the mountains east of the city. If I want heat, I can go to the desert. March came in chilly and struck a good note with me. I prefer cool over hot weather, and I got out and about with daily walks seven days a week.

Heather established herself early on in the month, when I was coming home from the grocery store carrying heavy bags and saw a pretty woman crossing the street in front of me. Heather said, "Yes, that Asian woman has a good figure, but what about *me*? You don't want that slant-eyed shit anyway."

I gritted my teeth and continued my walk, wondering if I could somehow not respond to her, and she'd shut up and go away.

"Has grit-and-grin *ever* worked for you?" she laughed. "You're fucking pathetic. I've been here ten years in your head, and you *still* haven't figured out a way to keep me out." She yelled over and over again, at the top of her lungs: "GIVE ME KIDS! COME TO L.A.! GET A GOOD JOB!"

She yammered on in this vein for days.

I went hiking with my friend Steve at a place called Iron Mountain, which is a moderate six mile hike over sometimes rocky terrain. The day was pleasantly cool, and I did my best to ignore Heather as she said things like: "That blonde has a nice ass, but would you want a girlfriend with a big dog?"

Steve and I reached the summit, where there was a telescope and some picnic tables. We sat down and ate sandwiches. Steve said, "This hike should make me tired, but I swim laps three days a week, and I'm in pretty good shape. Beyond that, it's all in the internal dialogue you tell yourself: 'The sun is not that hot, the wind is cool, I have good hiking books, and I'm having a nice sandwich here at the top of Iron Mountain.' Or you can say: 'I'm hot and sweaty, the wind blows dust to stick on my skin, it's hard on my ankles to scramble over these rocks, and I brought too much water so I have to carry that extra weight.' You choose how to frame the situation."

Heather said, in my mind: "Your friend prides himself on being upbeat. If he is *that* good at upbeat dialogues, why isn't he a billionaire? That's the goal the *real* geniuses of positive thinking set for themselves."

For a moment I thought it would be funny to tell Steve what kind of crap Heather said about him, but I could see that getting out of hand as Heather became meaner and meaner. So instead I ignored her, and she raised her voice: "Why don't you find a *female* hiking partner? You always hike with other men. How queer *are* you?"

If I ever find a hot female 'hiking companion,' I'll kick you out, I thought at her.

She went on to run down Steve's choice of clothes ("can we say, 'overdressed'?"), his lack of a hat on a sunny day ("fry his brain like an egg"), his rechargeable electric car ("cheap junk; the Japanese do it better"), his dog ("one foot in the grave, and not even pretty"), and his choice of hiking boots ("this is what you get from Chinese sweat shops").

These nasty little comments started to really grate on me, and I was not in a good mood as we went back down the mountain. My friend drove me to the nearest trolley station, where I hooked a ride back home.

On the trolley Heather went berserk: "That guy is UGLY!" she howled. "And that black lady, right there, have you ever seen such bug eyes? What about that kid—he speaks like a fucking retard… like YOU!"

I made it home and took off my hiking boots. I felt good from the exertion, and so I sent an email to my friend Daniel, suggesting we try something difficult, which was to hike El Cajon Mountain. According to what I had seen on the web, this is the hardest hiking trail in San Diego County. I was up for testing my mettle.

Daniel got back to me right away; he really liked the idea of taking on San Diego's most challenging hike. So we picked a day late in March and read up on the trail conditions, and I had something to look forward to other than the noise in my head.

Over the next few weeks, while I waited for the El Cajon hike, I read some books: *Happiness: A History, Creativity 101, The Truth is a Cave in the Black Mountains.* Heather's ongoing babble made it really hard to focus on reading, but if I read only about 40 pages a day, I could get away with it.

I have mentioned before that I did most of my useful activities in the mornings. Even in the bad cycles, I get a couple good hours a day. Encouraged by a week of good reading, I thought maybe I should try to write a short novel for 2016, but I thought that it would be a serious problem to write a novel with Heather antagonizing me. Even as I thought about this, the minor voices cranked up in a game of buzzword bingo:

"mumkin" *Maybe* I should marry Heather and give her kids. If, of course, I could find her to start with: tracking down hallucinations can be rough.

"heather" New messages from Heather coming soon.

"water"   These voices *seem* like an attack, but they're secretly giving me support. The more the voices hurt, the more support they were giving me.

"heaven" Once I give in and marry Heather, my life was going to be heaven, every day.

"everything" The voices need to steal everything in my mind, so they know me well enough to separate false from true and make me perfect in mind and spirit.

This sort of ongoing harassment occurred almost daily, and if there were reasons for breaks in the pattern, I couldn't discern them.

Around mid-month I went to the VA and met my new psychiatrist, who was pretty and young. I stared at her for a moment, hoping she knew her stuff, then she took me to her office. We went over my history and discussed my illness and its symptoms. Eventually she pointed out that the Seroquel didn't seem to help me much, and so she discontinued that and prescribed lithium, which is a mood stabilizer.

She said, "Let's give this a few weeks to take effect. Be aware of side effects, like frequent urination, tiring easily, or weight gain. Those are some of the common ones. If you experience *any* kind of pain or other extreme symptoms, call me right away."

So I started on lithium, but I knew it would take a month or even longer for it to kick in. I wanted to get rid of Heather, but I knew that most likely all that would happen is that she would be weakened a bit.

I mentioned in the chapter for February that I had developed a fascination with the homes of the rich and famous, especially the libraries of the well-to-do. I took the trolley to Heritage Park in the Old Town area of San Diego and looked at the Victorian houses there. These old houses, with their history of illustrious occupants, really hit my sweet spot, and of course I planned to buy one or more of them and have it moved downtown, or out into the neighborhoods closer to the mountains. You know, when the billion dollars came in.

Of course, Heather had to pipe up with: "These are drafty old termite-infested shit heaps. They're kind of pretty if you have no taste and can't think of anything better. America went through the Victorian era, and it's done with. And here it is, you could have a really great house, and you just want old crap. Just goes to show you, you're a dumb fuck."

As the interest in homes and remodeling pulled me one way, my genius infatuation pulled me another way. I read on the web that one of Albert Einstein's sons was schizophrenic and spent much of his life in asylums. Was that where I was supposed to end up, an asylum? Was Heather planning to drag me through the worst parts of my illness all over again, and I was going to be involuntarily committed? I read in the media that electroshock therapy was making a comeback in America, and the word was, some shrinks were using it on troublesome patients.

I got a small break from Heather around two-thirds of the way through March. I talked with my mother, and my father was not doing well. He had become so sick and weak that he could hardly get around at all, even in their house.

"These drugs the doctors gave him…these drugs are hard on a body," she said in a quiet tone. "They're especially hard on an *old* body. I don't know, Randal. He's really struggling. His doctor says it could go either way. Only the good Lord knows for sure what's going to happen."

She had been saying similar things for six months, and since there was nothing I could offer except moral support, I said, "Maybe this is just a little dip in a road that's going to head up to better places."

"We can only pray," she said.

News like this took me to a spiritual bad place that was like a black hole of worry where even Heather had no jurisdiction. My father had missed get-togethers with his siblings. He had missed hunting trips. He had been fighting cancer for two and a half years, and it was not clear whether he would win or lose. It *was* clear, however, that he was going to suffer along the way.

I had weird, disconnected dreams about my father, when I was a kid and he was much younger. This was probably in Muir Woods National Monument, a few miles north of San Francisco. I remember walking among the giant redwoods, smelling that rich forest smell and watching banana slugs slide along the wooden fences and leave their glistening trails of slime. In these dreams there were undertones of violence, that someone was coming after my dad.

Maybe the spirit of the forest had become angry because my dad had been a forester with the Bureau of Land Management for years and had approved permits for cutting trees.

This vague hint of karma made me unhappy, and I suspected Heather needled me in dreams that I could not remember. She had become so strong in my mind that she could even dictate the fates of my parents, or decide who suffered, and how long. Was she some kind of demon? Or dark angel? Or just a symptom of an illness that had more grip on me than I dared to admit to myself?

So I worried about my father's cancer, too.

The end of the month came up, and my friend Daniel and I took on El Cajon Mountain. This was a big, solid chunk of raw granite that you could see from miles away. From time to time I daydreamed that a dragon lived on top of the mountain. This was a huge dragon, thirty or forty feet long, and was of the friendly types, so long as you dropped at least ten dollars in coins onto its treasure heap. The dragon had a name, but I could never remember it. So I had fun with my imagination as Daniel and I walked the trail.

Good Lord, what a hike! About one mile into the uphill we ran into some guy in his thirties, dressed in exercise clothes, who looked half-dead. He was on the return journey, and he gasped at us: "The rangers need to post a sign that says: El Cajon Mountain, five miles uphill to the summit, and five miles uphill all the way back to the parking lot." He shook his head, drops of perspiration flying, and continued to stagger along.

He turned out to be right. The trail went up and down and up again, and just when you thought you were doing well, some smart aleck dumped a lot of gravel on the steep parts of the trails, so you constantly slipped and slid and fell on your behind. Under these circumstances it was very hard to maintain a conversation with my friend; I became so tired I couldn't even dream of dragons. On the up side, Heather couldn't get a word in edgewise, either.

It was five and a half miles to the summit, and when we got there we couldn't find the marker. So we tromped around a bit and sat on top of a boulder to take half an hour's rest.

The view was great, and we ate sandwiches and talked about the lowlands stretching out below us. I was hot, sweaty and tired, but we got a bit of a breeze, and that felt good.

Then we went back, another five and a half mile trek, and my whole body experienced pain the whole time. It really seemed that someone had tilted the trail so that we were actually going uphill when we should have been going downhill. The hike became miserable, and it seemed the sun became hotter as we made slow progress. I wasn't worried about water; I had half a dozen water bottles in my day pack, but I did worry about simply collapsing and being unable to move. By the time we were halfway back my hands and legs were trembling, and I felt wretched. My friend seemed to be doing better than me, but at one point he said, "Kind of a tough trail, isn't it?"

"A bit," I gasped. Then we got to a sign that said only one mile to go, and I knew it was mostly downhill. As the sun sank low we got back to the parking lot.

"That was not a fun hike," I said as we got into his car.

"I knew it was supposed to be tough," he said. "But now I can say I took on the hardest hike in San Diego County, and made it."

"I never want to hike this again," I growled.

"Come on, admit it, now that it's over, you had a good time. In fact, I feel so good, I insist we do it again next year."

"Fuck that," I grunted, and he laughed. He drove for a while and then dropped me off at my place, where the reward for the whole hiking trip was a hot shower and a good dinner.

For the next week, El Cajon Mountain haunted me. My feet were sore, my calves ached, and my legs in general continued to quiver. Getting out of bed was difficult, and I found it hard to stand up from a seated position because my knees didn't want to work.

But eventually I got over these signs of a tough workout, and I went back to walking every morning.

Heather returned as March slipped away. I was walking in Pantoja Park, which is a small, well-tended park on my daily walking route. It was about five-thirty in the morning and quite dark. There were some huge fig trees, and palm trees, and other trees I couldn't identify. A few homeless men slept on the grass, and I knew that pretty soon the sprinklers would kick in, and these guys were going to get drenched. I contemplated waking them up but figured this was a stupid thing to do. They could think I was a thief or rival homeless guy and pull a knife on me, or some such thing.

"You found my secret," Heather said, tossing her long auburn hair. She walked right alongside me, dressed in sun yellow top and jeans and tennis shoes; a marvelous hallucination and fully formed.

"You missed the hike up El Cajon Mountain," I said. There was no one in the park but the homeless guys. No one could hear me talk with Heather.

"No, I didn't *miss* it," she said with a sunny smile. "I was just wondering, why the hell did you climb such a monster mountain? Anyway, now you know that if you hike ten miles a day on impossible terrain, you can drive me off for a while."

I pondered this insight. Once I heard of a man who had crippling mental illness—I think it was bipolar disorder—and he couldn't work anymore and was in a bad way. When he had been younger, he used to run a few miles every day, but he had given this up as he hit middle age. Now, unable to focus because of his illness, and utterly without direction, he started running again just a few miles a day. And he noticed that the mental illness weakened. So he ran half a dozen miles a day. The symptoms weakened a little more. So he ran ten miles a day, and the symptoms went away.

Now he tried an experiment: he stopped running. Guess what happened? The symptoms came back. He was still ill, but running was a natural medicine for his body and mind.

So he said to hell with it, he was going to embrace this. He talked with nature outfits, and fitness gurus, and organizations dedicated to helping people with mental illness find recovery. And they sponsored him to go on runs wearing their logos and slogans. He wrote a book about his experiences, and he went on the radio and the internet and television to promote his healthy lifestyle.

And you know what? He's still running today, and his mental illness symptoms have been tamed.

I had sometimes gone hiking for ten miles, but I could not envision doing this every day. The inspirational story about this bipolar runner omitted the blisters and aches and pains, the wear and tear to his feet and knees and ankles, and those days when the exercise didn't help that much.

"If you would tone it down with the anger and the attacks, I wouldn't want to get rid of you," I told Heather, "But to answer your concern, I'm pretty sure that hiking or running ten miles every day isn't my way to cope. I need to work with my psychiatrist to get the right meds, and that takes noting my symptoms."

"Well, think fast," she said, "Because I predict that bad times are on the way."

Up Cycle

April: hypomanic showers…

The lithium caused nausea, and I hated taking the pills but knew if I didn't, the illness would become more intense. So there I was, bent over the toilet, my guts heaving, feeling awful but not able to throw up and get it over with. This was around the third of April.

"Good afternoon," Heather said cheerfully. "I see you're about to hurl, but I have a question for you."

I could not so much as move my head to see if she was visible, or if today she showed up as only a voice in my mind.

She flashed a series of half a dozen images of areas around San Francisco. I used to live in North Beach, and I liked to walk around that neighborhood and around other neighborhoods in The City. So there was an image of the inside of the local branch of the North Beach library, where I had checked out some books, and I saw Coit Tower, and the Marina Green, the Golden Gate Bridge, the twisty paths of Lombard Street, and so forth. With these memories came an intense longing to go back to San Francisco.

"Stupid mother fucker," Heather snapped. "You can't go back to The City. You don't have what it takes to live there."

I knew what she was talking about. San Francisco is very expensive, and I could no longer afford the cost of living there. San Diego is also pricey, but if you look around, you can find good deals on housing.

"San Diego has been good to me," I muttered, as another wave of nausea churned my guts.

"Ha ha ha, so cute!" she barked. "San Diego is good because I say it's good!"

"I took pains to make friends here," I said. "It's easy to find losers, but it's hard to find winners."

"Don't look now, but you've become a loser yourself."

She was right. I lived on next to nothing, could barely read, wrote only a small amount each day. I heard voices every day, and the medicines only partly controlled my symptoms. I longed for Heather to call off the assaults. Too proud to beg, I simply said, "We'll see what the new meds do."

"Yeah, they'll be *so* useful," she chortled. "That shrink of yours, she's wet behind the ears. Too young to know anything, too full of herself to listen to *you.*" Then she left me to throw up and feel terrible.

A few days after this I went hiking with my friend Steve at Los Penasquitos Canyon Preserve. The "trail" is actually a dirt service road that follows the south side of the creek through the preserve. There is a real dirt trail on the north side of the creek, and for the first few miles on the service road there are many trails meandering through the trees that line the creek.

After only a three mile hike, about halfway across the preserve, there is a small waterfall. There Steve and I ate sandwiches and drank some water, and I took off my shoes and went into the creek. The water was cold, and the shock of it on my legs was pleasant.

The return trip was not so nice. I kept thinking of San Francisco and the good times I had experienced there. I ran the Bay to Breakers once, which is a fun run all the way across The City, and once I participated in a marathon that went through a number of neighborhoods. Years ago I walked around some neighborhoods in The City, with a regular group of walkers, and I enjoyed seeing all the different architectural styles. I even once went on a volunteer event to clean up trash in Glen Canyon, which is a patch of wildlands set aside to give city dwellers a taste of nature.

With these memories came a tug of nostalgia. I had gone to college in San Francisco, many years ago, and I had stayed in The City for more than twenty years. But several of my favorite bookstores closed down during The Great Recession, and San Francisco didn't feel the same any more.

Back in the real world, Steve was in a hurry—he had some other event to head off to—and we hustled on the return trip. By the time we got back to his car I was surprisingly tired, and it felt like I had taken a much longer hike than I had.

Over the next few days, I had good energy. In fact, I had great energy. Instead of dreaming of failures and losses, I dreamed of dragons on El Cajon Mountain, and futuristic knights wearing powered armor. I remembered some of these dreams when I woke up, and I jotted down the basic outlines on 3x5 cards. As April went on, I filled up several such cards. Some of the ideas struck me as pretty good, and I discussed them with my friend Steve.

"Way to go," he said. "Are you becoming manic?"

I knew what he meant: typically I had maybe one or two good ideas for stories, each month. Now I has having one or two good ideas for stories, each *week*. But most of them I had when I was sleeping, or doing something else, and by the time I got to my cards, the ideas had slipped away. Who cared? I had so many ideas that I could afford to lose half of them.

"I'm *hypomanic*," I said.

"Keep it up," he laughed. "Maybe you'll get that killer idea that lets you break in to the pro level."

"Maybe," I said. We let the conversation stand there.

I had been writing stories and novels for 30 years, and some of my stories had been published in the token magazines and the semi-pro media, but breaking into the pros was a different matter. I had been trying for years, *decades,* with limited success. I read the web sites of famous fantasy writers. I read their how-to-write books. I looked up advice on the business side of writing, and on the editorial and agent aspects of the industry. What I ended up with was a mish-mash of often conflicting pieces of advice. Many professionals, though, said one thing over and over: write. Write short stories, write novels, write poems, but write and keep on writing. You'll never get anywhere if you don't produce work.

So I decided that I would write a new novel for 2016. I teased out the concept over a few days, and it turned out to be the sequel to another book I had written years ago. I did some research and jotted down an outline, figuring I'd start writing in May.

Heather showed up for a few hours a day, almost every day. "You're mentally ill because you left San Francisco," she proclaimed. "Money *doesn't matter.* You had tons of art and culture in The City. What do you have now?"

I have a strong writing group, and I've written some good stories here in San Diego, I thought back at her. *I didn't have that in San Francisco.*

"The City was better in every way," she said.

And that was the basic slant of our conversations. The minor voices chimed in like this:

"San Francisco rules"

"You're an idiot"

"San Diego sucks"

"Heather"

"art and culture"

"three kids"

"dumb ass"

As the month progressed, the ideas for stories just kept popping into my head. Most of these ideas I lost, because it's awkward to carry 3x5 cards into the shower, or write on them when you're using the toilet, and so forth. I had to set limits on how many random ideas I'd write down in a week, and that was two or three. It had been a long time since I'd been hypomanic, and I tried to enjoy it.

The thing is, when you experience a good flow of energy, it makes you feel great, and it helps you come up with ideas, but you become afraid that it's all going to go away. Hypomania never lasts that long; a few months is usually about it. So I was certain that this wasn't going to go on.

Unfortunately, Heather also rode the hypomanic wave. *She* was full of energy and used it to come after me in the shower: "Yo, moron, how about I sic the cops on you? You don't have enough challenges. Your life is like a bad story: no conflict, no reason to care about the main character." She stood on the other side of the shower door, so I couldn't see her, but her hands were on her hips, and I was sure she looked at me. "On the other hand, maybe not. Write the Great American Novel. Write something better than that. As for me, I think I'll destroy you."

It was right then, as Heather babbled and the hypomanic energy rushed through my nerves, that I realized the down cycle was over, and I was in an up cycle. It made sense. Heather was still there, but not as virulent or as insistent. It felt like I was able to work *with* my illness for my own betterment.

Up cycles tended to last a few months. I might get thirty or forty good story ideas, and of those, I might develop twenty ideas into stories. Unfortunately, hypomania was usually a precursor to full-on mania, so I had that to look forward to.

"I survived this down cycle," I said to her. "And I'll put this up cycle energy to good use."

"You'll get your ass kicked, and you'll fail," was her parting shot.

Heather's constant excoriation was not so hard to take now that my energy was high, but weird things started happening in the café, and I don't know to this day if they were Heather's fault or an expression of pure paranoia.

Around the halfway point in the month, I became convinced that all the people in the café were actors, saying their lines solely to drive home how vulnerable I was. These people weren't talking to me; they were sideways-talking, pretending to talk to others when actually their comments were meant for me. And at times, I was hearing statements I am pretty sure these people were not speaking. For example:

Black-haired young Asian woman: "He thinks he *owns* me. I

have to constantly guard boundaries with him. I think he flew the planes into the towers." Back to this again. 9/11, and was it a fraud? Had elites faked the whole thing and pocketed the money from the wars? Why wasn't anyone talking about this?

Middle-aged black man: "A bus goes by every ten minutes. You'd think, if you were doing badly in life, you could just jump in front of one of them." Was he speaking to Heather, or to me?

Young white mother with two little boys: "Two kids are a handful sometimes, but I'd still prefer three." I knew damned well who sent this 'message:' Heather.

White guy dressed like the season was winter: "The question is, what are you doing with yourself? Write, read, walk, and who cares? Who speaks for you? Who is on your side?" At that moment, it seemed I had no advocate, and overall I was not doing well. My mind was made up of gushing energy and weird ideas.

Middle-aged white guy looking homeless: "You'll never get rid of us. You'll have symptoms until you die."

Little black boy, with a smile: "Nobel Peace Prize is yours!"

Sometimes several symptoms hit at the same time, fueled by paranoia and attacks of fear. I would sit on my bed, reading the same paragraph a dozen times as the voices attacked. And this was an *up* cycle. This was an *improvement* over the last seven months.

Heather was apparently pleased with her earlier attacks, and so she started going farther back in the history of my schizoaffective disorder: "Good morning, douche bag. Do you ever wonder how your days full of voices and paranoia got started?" This was an afternoon near the end of the month of April.

"I suspect it was *you*," I growled.

"You brought it on yourself. You should have known from the first moment I started talking to you that something was really wrong. You should have gone to the shrink the very next day."

This sank in, and I said, "You're just a symptom, Heather. We have conversations as though you are real, but you're just a brain fart on steroids."

"Staying put was another mistake," she continued. "You should have left San Francisco a year earlier. Staying in The City was a costly, stupid mistake."

"I realized that," I said.

"You lived in a bedbug-infested, expensive SRO for over a year. Seven-fifty a month for a single room that overlooked a ventilation shaft? What a moron."

"I thought I'd get started again," I murmured. Her assaults were getting to me. "My delusions are to blame for a lot of that."

"The final blame is on you," she asserted. "Remember burning over a hundred thousand dollars back in 2007? Whose fault is that?"

This made me mad, but before I could say anything, she cut me off with, "We voices are stronger than you. We're smarter than you. We know what's real and what's not. You can't even find your meds without help, half the time."

Now she was simply making stuff up to needle me.

"9/11 was real," I babbled. Sometimes Heather could to this to me, could make me babble out loud. "I'm going to kick your ass," I snapped.

"How?" she said. "What exactly are you going to do?"

I started using my CBSST techniques and pictured people I cared about, and good times from my life. I hit her with this several times, over and over, and what the hell, after ten or fifteen minutes of fighting it out with her, I won, and she faded from my mind.

Over the last week of April Heather and I had a number of fights. Sometimes she won and made me feel stupid and guilty for all the mistakes I have ever made. She even brought up incidents from my childhood, like one from when I was seven and my little brother was about four. I was supposed to keep an eye on him, when we were playing in a field full of milkweed and monarch butterfly caterpillars, and instead I threatened to leave him there and go home by myself. He was pretty upset. As Heather brought this back, I felt unhappy with myself, and the question I had was, *how many of these incidents is she going to bring up? My whole life?*

I wanted to get up again, get going in life. I was 51 years old, I lived in a single room, and the only reason I had a shrink to rely on was because I was a veteran, with VA benefits. I had a small amount of disability money coming in each month. I spent most of every day fighting symptoms. Half the time I couldn't tell reality from delusions, and I felt deep fear of the cops, of the apartment manager, of Heather. Everyone was conspiring to keep me ill, so they could plot ways to take my money.

"Too wacko to be responsible with his own cash," said a minor voice, as the month came to an end. This was in my room, in the morning, as I wrote emails to friends.

"I've been keeping a budget my whole adult life," I said.

"Yeah, with occasional *excesses*," snickered another minor voice.

"I'll do *fine*," I said. "The financial problems are *your* fault."

"Give us all your money, or we'll hurt you," said a minor voice.

"Fuck you," I said. "I could get going again, if you bastards would just leave me alone."

I heard footsteps on the other side of the door of my room. One of the other residents on my floor had heard me talking with myself and had stopped to hear what I was saying. The front door was so thin that I could hear other people talking as they walked down the hall, and I knew those people could hear my mentally ill ravings.

I loaded a music CD into my computer and turned up the volume. The footsteps started again and went down the hall.

My relationship with the people on my floor was quite limited. In a Single Room Occupancy hotel such as the one I lived in, people came and went constantly. Most occupants rented a room for a few months, or six months at most, and then they moved on. So I didn't bother to learn their names and back stories. There were a few people who had been in their room a while, but it seemed foolish to try making friends among a transient population. You'd just get to know them, and *bam!* they moved on. I didn't know who wore the boots, but I didn't need word to go around that I was talking to myself.

May: ...bring story ideas

I remained hypomanic through May, and with the surge of pleasant energy came more good ideas for short stories about mental illness. These ideas I jotted down on 3x5 cards and filed for later use.

Some of the grand delusions that I had been suffering from, like 9/11 never happened or I will receive billions of dollars for good works I never did, backed down early on in the month, and they were replaced with much smaller delusions. For example, I was home in my room one day, and I was thinking about Heather and wondering why she wasn't bothering me. Immediately my computer made a chiming sound, and I "knew" that Heather was sending this chime to tell me she was watching everything I did on the computer. This was annoying and strangely comforting both.

You might wonder why it was somehow satisfying to hear from Heather. My friends had jobs, they were married; some of them had children. In short, they had busy lives. We emailed three or four times a month and talked on the phone once in a while. But Heather...she was there almost every day, for hours at a time. She knew everything about me: bad habits, good ideas, the miseries of mental illness. Even my closest friends didn't know me like she did. You'd think that with all the suffering she had brought to me, I would hate her, and sometimes I did, but she was probably the most reliable part of my life. I wouldn't say I "loved" her, but if she was gone for a few days, I started feeling anxiety that she was going to be gone for good.

One delusion of grandeur that kept going was this notion that I had convinced the Chinese military to withdraw from Tibet. The delusion kept recurring, like this: early in May I was looking for evidence that the Chinese really were pulling out. I looked on the internet, and some people were talking about their hopes that China would one day leave Tibet, but no one was saying it had actually happened. So I sat there, defeated, and then a minor voice said: "The peace process is fragile. But it is happening right now, and if you start raising a stink, you'll botch it all up."

"You guys said it was a done deal," I snapped.

"Work in progress," said the minor voice. "Let peace develop as it will. You're a hero: there are *billions* of people who admire you for this."

A second later, outside my room, a car horn honked. I blinked, and then I realized that the driver of the car was on my side for my role as peace maker. This of course meant that people could read my mind and honk that horn, all in less than two seconds.

So the sounds the computer made were messages from Heather and the minor voices, and just about anywhere I went the cars would honk their horns to show support for my good deeds. That is, deeds I could find no evidence for, no one talking about, and that were never mentioned by friends and family.

A week into the month I decided to put the hypomania to the test and started writing a new novel. It was going to be a story about a mentally ill man who goes up against a legendary ghost. This book was a sequel to my earlier novel, *Indian Spirits*, and it featured the same protagonist, who is a mentally ill man. I was excited by the story and wanted to see if I could trust hypomania to move me along.

So over the next few days I jotted down an outline, with the main bullet points of the story worked out, and then I sat down and started to write the book. I expected Heather to bother me a great deal, but she didn't. Not that day, and not for most of May. She still showed up from time to time, but she didn't aggravate me like she usually did. Somewhere around the tenth of the month she appeared as a voice in my mind:

"World peace, in your back pocket. Think you'll get any awards for that?" A car horn honked, off in the distance, just to reinforce her comment.

"Good morning, Heather," I said, slapping on a fake smile and figuring she was going to get ugly soon.

"I'm thinking about you," she said.

I gritted my teeth.

"My, so easily upset!" she laughed. "You've got this whole month planned out: your new book you want to write, some mental illness short stories to finish up, hiking with friends, and staying in touch with family. Just think, all that could go down the toilet at any moment."

My guts started to rumble, and I ran to the bathroom and got seated just in time.

I started employing CBSST techniques to get rid of Heather, and they actually worked. She lost her energy and faded to a minor whining in the distance.

My friend Steve also writes science fiction and fantasy stories, and he and I trade information on various articles we've read, web sites we've found, and interviews online, that offer ways to improve a writer's craft and market savvy. This is the same Steve who I have mentioned before as a hiking buddy. Unfortunately, the information you get from online articles often conflicts, and sometimes it is dated as well. So he and I discussed what strategies we were going to try, to get stories published and approach literary agents with finished works.

"I've found a professional map maker," he said with excitement. "I'm working hard on my novel, and I want a high-quality map. There's actually a web site for professional artists who have done maps for fantasy novels. I looked at the samples from various artists, and there's one woman who does really great work; when I think of a map for my book, it's her style I'm seeing. She doesn't come cheap: it'll be about $700 for an area map. I think it's worth it."

"Go for it," I said. My own personal economy didn't allow for expenses like $700 maps, but I was excited for him. We were both looking for a way into pro writing. For Steve, it was reading stories in pro magazines to see what other writers in the field were doing, and finding the latest advice from big names in the industry, and getting the best-looking map to accompany his novel. He figured, if you want to be a pro, study the pros and do what they are doing. Present yourself accordingly.

"I think my book is worth laying out some money," he said. "I have other ideas I want to pursue, too. Too early to make decisions; I'm just checking out what's available. Lot of self-published authors say it's important to write a good story, but you have to market it, too."

"I want to be a writer, not a salesman," I said. "But I no longer believe in this notion that the best stories get published. It's more like, the stories that tickle the editor's fancy at just the right time, on just the right day, are the ones that get into print."

That was where our conversation rested.

It's always a pleasure when I'm in an up cycle. Every decision I make seems clearer, and every day seems a little brighter and easier. One of the aspects of my illness that I don't mention often, because the delusions are much more interesting, is that my symptoms are often accompanied by *pain*. I get headaches from the attacks of the minor voices, like 'buzzword bingo,' and 'elimination,' and often there is a ferocious anxiety that comes along with Heather's put-downs. When I'm thinking ugly thoughts, like 'you should knock that lady down,' or 'throw that kid out in front of traffic,' I fear that Heather will get control of me, and I'll actually do harm to someone, or to myself. It hasn't happened yet, but she is in my mind most days, hours at a time, and that's a lot of time to pull off a coup.

In an up cycle, the amount of raw pain diminishes, and it's easier to tell delusions from reality. I spent more time trying to understand what had caused the last down cycle, and what made it so virulent.

All down cycles are bad, but at times there had been half a dozen symptoms going at once, and I had been a prisoner in my own psyche. Despite reading back through my emails and looking at what books I had been reading, I could not figure out what had triggered my illness. So I set this aside, in case Heather wanted to enlighten me at a later date.

At mid-month I walked to Balboa Park, which is the big central park in San Diego, and I passed by the museums and ended up at the Rose Garden. This collection of roses was in full bloom, and the blossoms were lively and colorful and wonderfully scented. I took pictures of a number of blooms, and I walked around the garden and sniffed the flowers, and when I was done I went home and sent the images to friends and family.

Something about this trip to the park felt great. May meant spring was in swing, and I felt excitement as I sent the images to the people I cared about. I hadn't even known San Diego *had* a Rose Garden until a Facebook friend posted a photo of it and prompted me to look it up. When I'm in an up-cycle, I can *live* again. I'm not just doing duty and taking care of my chores; I'm engaging with life.

Of course, hypomania often flares up into full-on mania, but I wasn't so concerned about that. I wanted to enjoy the days and the good mood I was in, and I could put up with the psychotic symptoms, in their reduced state.

In the mornings I kept up with my daily walks, enjoying the warm weather and staying in shape. People walked their dogs, and I took short forays into a small park on my walking route. The Parks & Recreation staff mowed the grass regularly and tended to the trees, and there was a scent to the park, of plants and sunlight, that I found pleasant. I was determined to stay in good physical health. My thoughts were often out of my control, but I could at least *feel* good by walking and hiking regularly.

Even in an up cycle, I couldn't just do anything I wanted. If I overdid an activity, the symptoms burst out again, so I had to take it easy. Just a few activities a day, and at a moderate pace.

One such activity was reading a fantasy book for children, entitled *Odd and the Frost Giants*. One of the features of the book was talking animals. In a weird flash of insight, I wondered why I had never had a conversation with an animal before? I had seen spirits during an earlier phase of my illness, and it seemed at times that pigeons or seagulls passed me messages, but they were not directly *talking* to me. And I hadn't come across discussion of other mentally ill people talking with animals, either. But the idea came from *somewhere*, and it has been a staple of stories for thousands of years. I'd bet that a mentally ill person was the first to think they could talk with animals.

So it was that I sent some finished stories to fantasy magazines, just to see if I could sell a few tales and make a little money. Maybe even break into the professional ranks. What could it hurt to try?

But most of my energy went to my new novel, which I titled *Weeping Woman*, and I sat down early each morning and wrote 1,000 words for the book. This may sound like a lot, but there are writers out there who write a million words a year. A *million*. I was aiming for 95,000 words with my book, so it was a joke compared to these prolific writers. But given my illness, that seemed like plenty to accomplish. That is, 10% of what the big boys were writing. On more than one day I sat there in front of my computer, cursing my illness and Heather and wondering what I could accomplish if I was not weighed down with schizoaffective disorder.

"If only these people would stop knocking me down," I complained to my closest lady friend, Jackie. She and I are both mentally ill, and we both read fantasy novels. We had an ongoing email conversation.

It was late in the month when the rejection emails started coming in from the magazine editors. Most were form letters that told me nothing, but a more useful rejection read like this: "The main character seems real, and you've drawn realistic scenes, but somehow the story fails to totally engage me. It's not quite what I'm looking for at this time."

"Who is knocking you down?" Jackie asked me. "Heather?" I had told her all about Heather.

"These people in the café, and the homeless on the streets. The cops, too. It seems like *everybody* is in on it."

"Am I in on it?" she asked.

Heather broke in, a faint hallucination that was more felt than seen, and she laughed until her face was pink. "Jackie *leads* the attack team!"

"Yes!" I blurted. "She's talking right now."

"To hell with her. I'm talking with you, too. Ignore her, and maybe she'll go away."

"Now it's the magazine editors, too. They say good things about my writing, but they don't *buy* the stories."

"That's because you're a shitty writer," Heather suggested.

"Because all these people are reading your mind and saying ugly things that weaken you?" asked Jackie.

"Yes. I might not ever have been mentally ill. It's just these constant attacks: people running me down, people repeating the same big promises and telling me I have all these skills I don't actually have. *They* are the ones who make me crazy."

"But that's gotten quieter now, you said."

"You know what the scariest part of that is? Knowing that almost for sure the fires of mental illness will blaze bright again in a few months."

"You know," she said, "It's possible to cause bad things to happen, by thinking about them too much."

"I'm trying to enjoy this slack time, but it's the sensation of seeing that light farther down the tunnel. It's almost certainly a train, and when it finally gets here, the impact is going to *hurt*."

"I think your symptoms *reflect* your illness; they don't *create* it."

"I can't tell which causes what," I said. "Be glad you don't have psychotic symptoms; now *that* is crazy."

Heather butted in with, "Why don't you tell her, 'Jackie, you're an ugly bitch, and I hope you drop dead.'"

I gritted my teeth and ground out, "Jackie, I have to go. Heather wants in on our conversation, and once she starts she won't stop."

"Tell her she's nothing but a symptom, and one day you'll make her go away."

"Tell her that she can—" Heather started, but I pictured myself hiking Iron Mountain, and that CBSST substitution worked. She said a few ugly things and then went away.

By the last week in May I was feeling stronger and more stable. I wondered what was happening with the lithium: was this drug the reason why I was having weak symptoms, or was I in a natural up cycle? lithium is a mood stabilizer; it wouldn't go after Heather or the other psychotic symptoms directly but would even out my emotional imbalances. That is, I *hoped* that was what it would do.

As a result of the good mood and more restful nights I was experiencing, certain errant thoughts began floating through my mind. Like, *what if the psychosis is caused by excessive emotions? Get control of the moods, and the psychosis goes away. This may be the beginning of the end, but not* my *end—Heather's.* I was afraid to hope, because I had been through up cycles before, and things improved for a while and then got worse again. My expectations did not seem to have any effect on what really happened.

Buoyed up by the hypomania, I began thinking about work. My hobbies—writing stories, reading books, hiking—didn't bring in any real amount of money. I only pursued them a few hours a day, and the rest of my day I walked around my neighborhood, listened to music, and took naps.

It was possible that this up cycle could be the last of my mental illness. The lithium might finish it off and allow me to come back to life. There were two roads in front of me: assume the up cycle would go on another month or two, until all the symptoms ended and I became well again, or assume that bad times would return once more, and the up and down cycles would go on for only God knew how many more years.

Because I was hypomanic and had a flow of good energy going, I figured I could beat my illness. I felt this way during every up cycle, and this time I gave into it again. I started looking at job listing sites on the web, and one of my weekly chores became looking for work. I wasn't sure what kind of work I could do, given that I sometimes talked to Heather out loud, or experienced minor voices harassing me, and so forth. A big part of me wanted to give up before I had even started, but the hypomania urged me onward.

What could possibly go wrong?

June: dad's birthday

The answer to the question of what could possibly go wrong came early in June, when my gentle hypomania turned into the nasty, head-on mania that I had feared. My energy went out the roof, and I started buying things. All of a sudden I "realized" I needed a new web site, and I needed to buy more books, and of course summer was imminent, so I needed new shorts and t-shirts. I spent hundreds of dollars I didn't really have, so I figured what the hell, I'll put it all on plastic!

My days became a back-and-forth battle between trying to control my spending and finding new things to want. In absolute terms, I was spending small amounts of cash. But in terms of my personal budget, wasting four hundred dollars in a single month was a disaster. My disability income was a lot less than two thousand dollars a month, and here I was chewing through a quarter of my entire income on frivolities. Because of this, I started having bad dreams in which I ran out of money and became homeless.

Anxiety attacks came and went as I wondered how I would ever get back on track financially. Every time I resisted a purchase, the money I saved seemed to burn a hole in my pocket. I just *had* to have a new business suit, and even more books, some pieces of art to decorate my room, and rich foods to eat. Some of you who are reading these words probably know the crazed spending that comes with mania.

I had an appointment with my shrink, and she asked how my symptoms were. I told her I was having a hard time controlling spending, that I was now in full-on mania.

"I'd say it would be a good idea to try the lithium a little longer," she said. "It really is effective for many people."

"I think lithium reduced my symptoms," I said. "I *should* be totally out there, but the drug reduced the attack to hypomania for a time. Yes, I want to stick with it for a while and see if it gets control of the affective symptoms."

So that was what we did.

With the hypomania gone to full mania, the story ideas I had been having dried up. I had lots of energy, but it expressed itself as jumbled thoughts and spikes of pain when my mind was filled with calls for urgent action. One of the worst symptoms was not being able to sleep at night. I woke up every half hour, full of manic energy, and when I could not go back to sleep, I tossed and turned for another half hour. I had not experienced these symptoms in a long time, and I didn't like them. But what could I do but take the lithium and wait for it to control the illness?

"Why do you exercise *every goddamned day*?" Heather snapped, as I went on my morning walk. "It's not going to make me go away."

"Nobel prize," said a minor voice.

"China out of Tibet"

"Middle East peace"

"worth billions"

At this point you may reasonably ask, other than the manic spikes and the money wastage, what changed? It's the same old voices, saying the same old things as the days heated up and summer arrived.

"Every shrink I've had has recommended regular exercise," I growled at Heather. "I *like* to stay in shape."

"You're going to die one day like everyone else. Exercise won't save you from death."

"But I might get five or ten years more life," I said. "And *healthier* life; not hooked up to a fucking oxygen tank."

"Okay, Randy. Whatever you say." She farted, just to be disrespectful. I noticed the familiar form of my name, and as I walked past a hotel, with people near, I thought, *Why 'Randy'?*

"You haven't earned anything better. You're like a child; all you're worth is a slice of your full name. You have to *earn* the rest."

This made no sense to me, and by the time I got home, I had all but forgotten Heather's nonsense.

In the spirit of enjoying exercise, I went with my friend Daniel and his wife and young daughter and hiked Cowles Mountain, which is a short hike and not too steep. It took a long time to get to the top, with a seven-year-old kid along, but the view from the summit was great, and we ate snacks and took some pictures to capture the experience.

"When you get older, you can hike in the forests," I said to my friend's kid. "These little shrubs in San Diego are good, but Big Sur is better, or Sequoia National Park, or Muir Woods."

"I don't *like* hiking," she grumbled, as we followed the trail back down the mountain.

"It's easier when you're an adult," I said. Immediately I thought of the punishment Daniel and I had experienced hiking El Cajon Mountain, and that shut me up for a few minutes.

"You did well on *this* hike," Daniel said.

"It's hot," she complained.

"We got to see the mountains," said her mom.

The girl didn't answer. I wondered how many of these lessons we were trying to share with her would stick. I was a believer in nature, had been since I was a kid. I thought my goddaughter spent too much time watching movies, but how could I point this out without her parents saying in return, that I read too much?

"I hate hiking, too," Heather complained. "You know, you should slap your god-daughter. Just punch her in the face."

This wasn't the first time Heather had urged me to hurt someone, but as we hiked down off the mountain and my friends took me home, Heather said, "Or rape someone. That would be bold. You should try new things from time to time."

Fuck off, I thought at her.

She retaliated by singing *The Star Spangled Banner*, off key and ugly. Then my friends dropped me off at my building, and Heather seemed satisfied. She was quiet after that.

I asked before: what about my illness changed? For starters, Heather wasn't as loud, and when she did show up, she didn't stay as long. The minor voices didn't come around as often. The lithium and the manic spikes fought it out, and the mania stabilized at an intensity that I could handle. All my symptoms were a bit more muted, and I could carry on with activities I enjoyed.

A few delusions of grandeur continued, as I've noted, but I had more mundane delusions as well. Every time I saw cops in a patrol car, I thought they were going to plant drugs on me, and their crony judges were going to give me twenty to life in the War on Drugs.

For some reason the apartment manager featured in a number of paranoid delusions. I thought he was going to let himself into my room and steal my computer, or cut my throat while I slept.

There was no real reason for any of these delusions; I was not wanted by the police and had not had a quarrel with the apartment manager. This was simply the illness making itself felt.

There were hallucinations as well. I saw bugs crawling on my computer, but nowhere else. I came close to these 'insects,' and instead of scurrying off, they simply disappeared, which is how I knew they were a hallucination.

Once, when I was seated in front of my computer, I heard a sound like the beating of pigeon wings. A bright light gleamed from my refrigerator. The fridge had been running loud for a while, and I figured it was going to stop working, and I'd have to buy a new one.

Instead, the door opened, and an angel stood there, about two feet tall, just small enough to fit inside my mini-fridge.

Fool, the angel said. But it didn't speak; it was projecting its thoughts to me. *You are slipping.*

What do you mean? I thought.

But the angel was content to give me a worried look, and that made me wonder what was wrong. Was the angel telling me I was slipping because of my delusions, or was I slipping in a spiritual way? Was I going to have a spiritual crisis? What would that entail?

The angel spread its wings and flew up into the ceiling. But the thought that I was about to have an emotional or spiritual crisis stayed with me.

Around two-thirds of the way through June, Heather showed up, standing in the café while I read a book and drank a cup of coffee.

"Hey, Russell, how's it going?" she asked.

I didn't look at her and waited for the cruel comment, slur, or running-down that she usually did. I remembered that she was doing something with my name, calling me wrong names or some such crap to needle me.

"You know," she said sharply, "You're not a bad guy, when you listen to others. It's when you go it alone, without me, that I don't like you."

This was unusual, and I glanced over at her, to where she wore a black and yellow running suit and running shoes. Her hair was held back behind her head somehow, and she had rosy cheeks as though she had been exercising for a while. She was very pretty, and I looked around the café and saw a dozen people. So instead of talking I thought, *What do you want, Heather?*

"Why do you think I called you 'Russell,'?" she asked.

I don't know. I don't care.

"See, you're being a dick again. Don't people frequently call you 'Russell'? People who don't know you well? So I called you 'Russell,' because you don't know your own future. Look out the front window of the café. What do you see?"

I turned in the chair and saw a police car going past.

"Those guys are going to kill you one day," she said in a pleasant tone. I glanced at her and saw that she still had rosy cheeks, but her eyes shone bright green and cold.

I think enough Americans kill each other, there's no need for any more, I thought. This was just an off-the-cuff comment, and her response was to walk out the front door of the café and disappear.

On my dad's birthday I called to see how he was doing, and he said, "Glad to hear from you. Things are as good as I can expect. I feel weak, all the time; nothing new there. It's really hard to get up and around. We were thinking about going out to a Mexican place for birthday dinner, but I don't think I'm going to be able to do that. It's all I can do to sit and read a book. Let's not talk about what it's like to have to go to the bathroom."

We talked a while longer, and then I let him go, rather than wear him completely out with too much conversation.

This chat with my dad got me thinking about diseases of the body versus diseases of the mind. His cancer made him weak, and the pain of the disease, and the chemo, made it hard for him to concentrate. My schizoaffective disorder made me mentally weak, and I too had a hard time concentrating. Was it natural to compare and judge who had the worse condition? But at least his mind was sharp; how many pages a day was he reading, as opposed to my lousy forty pages a day?

Then I realized that the angel I had seen was probably connected to my father's ongoing illness. When I thought back over the progression of his cancer over the last three years, it was slowly wearing him down. He had needed surgeries to remove infected lymph nodes, and he needed chemotherapy, and even as he fought, he had to stop taking daily walks, and he had to sleep more hours a day and felt tired even when he was awake. The situation was like watching two heavyweights beating each other bloody, and not being able to guess which one would win.

To me, the angel hallucination meant an emotional crisis. I *worried* for my dad, but the catch-22 in the situation was that if I called frequently to see how he was doing, I would only tire him out faster and make him more vulnerable than he already was. It was sad that he could not even manage to find enough strength to go out to a restaurant with my mother, for his birthday.

Beyond that, how many more birthdays did he have left?

Heather came back, this time when I was in the shower, and she wore a sky-blue bikini. "I like seeing you this way, Randolph," she said.

"Randolph?" I grumbled.

"'Randolph' kind of sounds like your name, but it isn't really you," she commented. "Not as far off as 'Russell,' but still not together yet. So come on, get it together. Beautiful young woman just waiting for your touch. That could be the *real* you. Mentally ill loser, all alone? Is that you? What would it take to change that? Where do I find 'Randal?' Think about that. Think about what it would take to be a *winner*."

"I have several friends who are 'winners,'" I mumbled. "I don't want to figure out how to be some mini-me. I want to be myself, and maximize myself."

She laughed. "You're a winner, to me. It's just that you're so wrapped up in your pitiful little life that you barely know I'm here."

I tried to pin her in my gaze, but she became a mere voice in my head, and the harder I concentrated, the more she hid herself. "What do you want, Heather?" I asked. Compliments were rare, and there was no way she was offering support with nothing in return.

"Come to Los Angeles," she said, suddenly earnest. "We'll snuggle in together, and the people running your show will give you your money. And your awards. And everything you're due."

She didn't swear, or use slurs, or run me down. In fact, she sounded more than reasonable; she sounded *nice*. I shampooed my hair and turned off the water and toweled dry. A few minutes later I returned to my room. She was up to something, that was clear. Or I had just reached a major milestone in my illness, and everything was up for grabs.

"I'll think about it," I muttered, and outside the building, a small dog barked.

Every few days I had paranoid delusions about run-ins with the cops. In these fantasies, the police arrested me at the café, so all the patrons would see me perp-walked to the patrol car and shoved in like a prisoner. The cops were going to take me to jail and book me in. They put me in a large holding cell and took my cuffs off. There were half a dozen rough-looking men in the cell, who appeared to be homeless people.

"Give him a big welcome," said one of the cops, then he shut the metal door to the cell.

The six men promptly beat the hell out of me, then one of them tapped on the door. The cop came back and pulled me out of the cell, put chains on me, and hauled me through the streets of San Diego, where everyone saw I was a prisoner.

"I'm innocent!" I yelled, and the cop punched me in the chest. I couldn't get draw breath, and I staggered along.

"None of that nonsense," said the cop. He led me to an empty courtroom, where there were no attorneys or witnesses or supporters. There was just the judge, who was a middle-aged black man in the traditional black robes.

The cop dragged me up to stand before the judge.

"This fine officer has found anti-psychotic drugs in your possession," said the judge.

"I'm mentally ill," I protested. "I *have* to take pills."

"You're a head case," said the judge, and he lifted his gavel. "Guilty of harboring mental disorders. Mental illness is a crime in America. I sentence you to twenty years in the prison-industrial complex. That will be all." He brought the gavel down hard, and in that loud *whack* I thought my very soul shattered.

The fantasy ended at that point. There was not a single one of these delusions; there were several of them, *every day*. Cops were out to kill me. Cops and judges were out to frame me. Cops killed someone and blamed me for the crime. Homeless people plotted to kill my friends and finger me.

I was of the opinion that *something* triggered these symptoms, but it could be an article in the media that I'm thinking about, or a remark from passersby that I overheard, or a comment from friends and family, or who knows what. Half the time the symptoms seem like the random firings of my brain as it accesses old memories to build a framework for events in the here and now.

I thought I should take advantage of this up cycle and look for a job, and I even went as far as to look online for positions, but every time I thought about it, I mulled over these paranoid delusions, and I thought about Heather going on for hours and distracting me from whatever I was trying to do, and I thought about how am I going to stick to a task if my head is filled with voices, and so forth. At times I got into verbal quarrels with Heather, and how would that look to my colleagues?

Continuing with those thoughts, what employer would let me work half days, taking advantage of the fact that I was clearer in the mind in the mornings? And when the up cycle was over, and bad times returned, I would need to either be granted unending understanding of why I was such a mess and barely able to complete my tasks, or I would have to quit work for the duration of the down cycle and wait for better symptoms to return.

When I thought of the situation like this, I would clearly be a fool to look for work. I was going to have to limp on with my current situation, looking for ways to improve my lot in life. There was no way I could count on the illness to suddenly come to an end.

"It's all up to *you*," Heather babbled happily.

I sat at my computer and closed the job search tabs I had opened.

"If it was up to me, I'd have been well years ago," I muttered.

"You *like* being sick, I think," she said. Now, normally she would have needled me with this, but she was back to her nice tone again.

"You mean I *like* nausea from the lithium," I growled. "I *like* voices cutting in when I'm trying to read a book, and their making big promises that are never realized? I *like* being afraid every time I go outside, that the cops or the judges or the politicos have it in for me?"

"You have to *fight*," she said. "Keep switching drugs. Do more exercise; do harder hikes. Knock off with all the potato chips and dip. You're drinking a glass of red wine every day…"

"That's supposed to be good for my heart," I said.

"Cocaine is supposed to be good for your self-confidence, too," she jabbed. "Self-serving baloney. Get healthy. Get well."

"If I get well, what happens to you?" I asked.

"There are many paths in life, and they all lead to Heather. Got it, Randy?"

I didn't respond, and I guess that means she won the fight. She left, and I felt a fierce sense of loss that was almost heartbreak. Was there any way to get over schizoaffective disorder? Or was I going to drag on like this for the rest of my life?

July: Heather

My minor delusions seemed to proliferate as July rolled in. One morning I got out of bed around 4:00 am and mumbled to myself, "I need to get a job." This, in spite of the fact that I had already decided not to continue looking for work.

Immediately, a small dog barked outside. Then two or three large dogs took up an excited barking. This was a conversation: the small dog was me, suggesting ways to better myself within my limited resources, and the big dogs were the politicians, Hollywood executives, and New York media moguls who were actually in control of my destiny. I went to the window and looked out on the street, and no dogs were in view. Real barking? Imaginary yapping? Or pure hallucination? Take your choice.

I dressed, picked up a book and went to the café for a cup of coffee and what I hoped was the silent companionship of other patrons who were up this early. Instead, Heather said, "Bet you can't find me, Steven."

Bet I'm not even going to look, I thought. *Bet I don't respond to 'Steven.'* Steven was my middle name.

"You know where I live," she said. "Come find me, and make me stop calling you names."

I glanced around the café and didn't see her; apparently this visitation was just a voice, no image. *You're being nice lately,* I noted.

"And yet you are all worried and anxious that I'm here to hound you. Have I *ever* given you a hard time?"

This question was so ridiculous that I couldn't even address it.

A white guy who looked homeless—tattered and dirty clothes, red face, wild hair—shuffled past the front windows of the café.

I thought, "*I'm not going to Los Angeles to look for you, Heather.*"

The homeless guy dropped a beer bottle, which hit the sidewalk and made a loud sound of ringing glass. I knew without Heather saying a word that this sound meant 'recycle.' She was going to bring up this idea of going to L.A. again.

"Gosh," she purred, "I sure would like to have three kids with you. You're my kind of man, Steve, even as far off the mark as you are today. I'm not *harassing* you. The cops *harass*. I'm just a poor little journalist…who is in love with the wrong guy?"

I sat there, amazed, wondering what she was up to now. 'In love'? She had never used language like *that* before.

What is happening with you? I thought at her.

She sniffled a little bit, as though she was crying, and made no more comments. I went back to reading my book and took to glancing out the windows as I looked for cops on their way to put me in jail.

Over the next week I went about my usual rounds. I read a little and wrote a little every morning, and went out for a coffee, and walked a mile and a half to stay in shape. But I was not alone during these activities: no, sir. I lived in the presence of my imaginary girlfriend, day after day.

As the weather got ever hotter, I tried to spend more time indoors. And she was waiting for me. Two young women in the café were talking one sunny afternoon.

"Do you think she's going to be promoted?" asked one young woman.

"She is the best choice in the department," said the other.

I glanced at these women, who were dressed in frilly dresses to take into account the heat, and as they said, "she," Heather appeared. She wore a frilly summer dress, too, thin and almost see-through, with blue and white patterns that somehow looked upscale to me.

"So glad to see you," she said to me. "You should talk with these girls. Get them to lay you. Try a threesome. Wouldn't that be fun?"

I thought. *You usually get mad if I even look at another woman.*

"It's summer, you shouldn't be lonely. See how reasonable I can be?"

When am I going to get my money? And what about the Nobel Prize?

"You keep returning to these two, more than the other awards you're due. Trust me, when you get that Nobel, your bed will be filled with women. If that's what you still want. Remember that it takes several years to go from being listed for the Nobel, to winning it."

I've suffered enough for a dozen prizes, I growled.

"Steven, *everyone* suffers a little now and again. Immigrants suffer, refugees suffer; misery never ends. You hear? You need friends."

I have friends.

"Come to Los Angeles and knock me up. Pretty, pretty please?" She smiled a stunning grin. Really, she was beautiful in that moment, and a sense of uneasiness gripped me.

Are you in an up cycle, too? I asked her, unnerved by this change.

She shook her hair, and then she disappeared.

Days later I was at the library, reading some poetry out of a book. I had a chair in front of the plate glass windows, and some voices interrupted me. In the stacks behind me, a woman talked with a teenage boy. I didn't turn around to see these people; I just heard them talking.

"All these books are *foreign* books," the young man said in disgust.

"They're translations into English," said the middle-age woman. "What are you looking for?"

"Were are the books by men?" asked the teen. "I want to read something like a sword fight, or hunting lions. Maybe a bullfight, in Spain. Stuff like that. But I don't know the titles to look for."

"Sounds like you might enjoy Ernest Hemingway. He was into sport hunting and that type of thing."

"Great! Is he here with these books?"

"No, different section. Come on, I'll show you."

And as soon as the two people stop talking, Heather was there. No visuals this morning, just her saying to me:

"Poetry? Since when do you go for that?"

"I read poetry from time to time. Robert Frost, Martin Espada, Ogden Nash." All this, muttered so no one in the stacks could hear me.

"There are more important things to do with your time than read a silly poem about a zoo."

"Like what?" I mumbled, expecting more talk of moving to L.A.

"Some friends of mine are coming to visit you soon. You must treat them with respect."

I turned around in the chair and looked into the stacks, but there was no one near. So it was okay to talk closer to regular volume.

"You mean, in my head?" I said with heat. "More goddamned voices?"

"That's not *respect*," she snapped.

"If you want me to be nice, go away and find someone else to fuck with," I suggested.

There was a long pause, several minutes, and I read another poem.

"Let me show you something," she said, and a grainy black-and-white image of several dirty, half-starved children and a desperate-looking woman appeared in my mind. "The speakers for the left say, 'help these poor people get food and shelter.' They call this 'compassion,' but they may mean 'class warfare,' with the rich taxed to pay for the upkeep of the poor."

"And?" I asked.

"Given their way, they'd tax the hell out of everyone and give trillions of dollars to the indigent."

"I'm in the mood for poetry, Heather, not a political discussion."

"Discussions may come to you, though, and it would be a wise decision to hear me out, because I might be the clearest, best choice you have, in the future."

She didn't dig at me, or criticize me, or terrorize me, or even use harsh language. My time with the book of poetry was clearly over, and a sense of unease rippled through my guts.

An image of an ICBM roaring out of its silo flashed in my mind, and Heather said, "The right claims we need more nukes and more guns and more soldiers, planes, tanks, napalm, and more nationalism and xenophobia to fuel all the weapons of war. This vision also requires trillions of dollars."

"And you want me to take sides," I said.

"What is the difference between the left and the right, if they both have tin cups in hand and are begging for money?"

"You mean in methodology, or what?" I grumbled. She had not said anything ugly or cruel, but I felt badgered nonetheless.

She drove on: "I'd argue that the basic stance of the left is 'compassion,' and the basic stance of the right is, 'belligerence.'"

"And *I* would argue that a country needs both," I said.

"Which side *do* you take?" she asked primly.

"I just took it."

"The right are a pack of thugs and murderers," she said, and I froze in the chair, afraid I had spoken her words out loud. "Remember that article you read, that mentally ill people are sixteen times more likely to be killed in an encounter with the cops, than regular people? What does that mean, for you? Think about it."

I sat there, the book of poetry in my hands, as I took in these ideas. If the right was murderous, and if the cops were on the right, and if the cops were gunning for me just because I was mentally ill…

Then at some point I had to become murderous, too, or they'd get me first. But I was not prepared to hold onto this idea, and as I went back to reading amusing poems about zoo animals, Heather and her politics disappeared from my mind.

On the fourteenth of July I bought a bottle of wine and a wedge of cheese and sat in front of my computer at home. I looked up the online obituary for a lady friend of mine, named Nina. I met this woman in 2008, at the community mental health center in Santa Fe, New Mexico, where we were both getting treatment for our mental illnesses. I was blazing schizoaffective, and she had been severely depressed for years. We formed a loose friendship, based mostly on the fact that she made fun of those of us who heard voices. Eventually she was awarded disability and found an apartment, and I got onto disability and moved back to California. A few years passed, and I decided to look her up. I didn't have her current contact information, so I got in touch with a mutual friend, who told me:

"Nina is dead, Randal. I'm sorry. She died a few years ago, in a traffic accident. There was an article in the paper, look up her name and you'll find the story."

I looked up the article, and there it was: she and a friend had been standing at a crosswalk, waiting for the light to change. This was early evening, and it had been dark. For some reason my friend ran out into the crosswalk and was hit by a truck and killed instantly. The day she died was July 14. Maybe I've been lucky so far, but I have not had any friends die except this gal. So she gets her own day, where I celebrate her life and that six months or so when we shared some laughs and pondered whether or not we were going to ever beat our illnesses, or if they'd beat us.

I think it likely, based on comments she had made from time to time, that her depression beat her. It wasn't hard putting myself in her shoes: years of feeling bad *all the time*, living at poverty level with all the problems that come with that, thinking again and again of putting an end to the ongoing pain...until running in front of a truck seemed like the best choice.

She had been around my age, and her death really bothered me. I poured wine and drank up, and I nibbled the cheese down to nothing. I could picture her running out into the road and embracing the ongoing truck. The news article even mentioned which specific intersection she died in; I have walked across that street myself and had been dismayed at the speed of the oncoming traffic.

Finally the wine was gone, and I was buzzed, but I had an insight into my friend's death and why it caused me such sorrow. She was the only individual that I had known personally who had probably died of mental illness. And of course, if mental illness could kill her, it could kill *me*. All my symptoms, and the sheer tenacity of the disease over a long time, meant I too was in the cross-hairs.

Heather did not come around during my celebration of Nina's life. It was hard for me to believe, but she didn't show up or even put in some words for or my friend.

Outside my window, someone dropped a glass bottle on the sidewalk, and it made a loud sound as it bounced off the concrete. Either my dead friend or Heather was going to be recycled, and soon.

Cameras. The damned things were everywhere: at the grocery store, in the library, and even monitoring the apartment building where I lived. It was clear that someone was spying on me, and either Heather or the government was in on it. Some day they were going to have the special effects guys in Hollywood dummy up some damning video images that made me look like a criminal. After that, it was all a done deal: off to prison for the rest of my life.

What were they going to accuse me of? Kicking someone's dog out into traffic? Threatening a pedestrian's life with a letter opener?

Once upon a time I owned a nine millimeter pistol, and the cops seized it during a random stop-and-search.

"The cops kept your gun," Heather said forcefully. She was just a voice in my head; no visuals this time around. "Guess what? It's going to show up again, associated with you. Fancy being pegged as a murderer?"

This scared the hell out of me, because the media ran frequent stories about cops planting drugs on people, or in their homes and businesses. And it seemed incredible, but a lot of people serving on juries thought that planting evidence was good police work! So not only did cops plant evidence, they got away with it.

What chance did I have if the cops came after me? Heather could tell them every bad decision I have ever made. This situation was very bad, and I didn't know what to do about it. So I dithered, and the parade of days continued.

On my birthday, late in July, I went to a restaurant and had a very tasty seafood dinner. The best part of it was a salmon steak that was done just right. I shelved the worries about the police and surveillance cameras and a vengeful Heather, and I just ate. Because it was the height of summer, the day was hot, but there were umbrellas over the tables. Those created some refreshing shade.

I decided to try focusing on something other than cops and guns and planted evidence, so I counted my blessings:

- My family and friends were supportive of my hobbies and the positive activities in my life
- My symptoms hadn't killed me yet
- I could hike, and walk, and read and write a little each day
- I had survived more than a decade of schizoaffective disorder
- There was enough disability money each month that I could celebrate my dead friend's life or go out to eat at a restaurant for my birthday

When I looked at my situation from this angle, my life wasn't all bad. That of course got me thinking of symptoms and all that came with my illness, and it seemed to me that the negative aspects of my life were a sea, and the positive aspects were a little boat that kept me from drowning. It was a sobering way to look at my life, and I finished my dinner and paid my check in a serious mood. I imagined that my friend who had died must have done the same reckoning that I had just gone through, and she found no boat to keep her above water.

During the last week of July, I saw an article in the local paper, about an ambush on a police foot patrol. One officer had been killed, and another had been wounded. The police spokesman didn't know if this attack was related to other attacks on police that had been going on across the country, or if this was an isolated incident.

In response to this news, I took a walk up to police headquarters, a few blocks away from my building. On the north side of the building I found a granite memorial to fallen officers, festooned with bouquets of flowers.

My relationship with the police was complicated. I was taught, growing up, that one respected the police and the law they represented. But it seemed the media was full of stories of cops blowing away unarmed black men, or cops accused of rape and other criminal activities. The citizens were getting tired of it, and some were fighting back. Were these people outlaws? Mere criminals? Or were they a sort of freedom fighter, where oppressed minorities drew blood for blood? And how much of this was spin and nonsense?

I snapped a few pictures of the monument and returned to my room, where I sent the pictures and well-wishes to a friend of mine who is married to a police officer. She thanked me for the kind words, and I was left feeling torn. Good cops, bad cops. Supporters of the police said that most cops are good cops, doing a hard job, and most citizens are honest people who don't hurt anybody.

All these ideas, these positions, these stances, seemed equally valid to me. The cops killed citizens; citizens kill the cops. Families in both camps suffered, and no one knew how to end the violence. Bottom line? All's fair in love and war.

Heather had missed a few opportunities to hit me when I was weak, but that didn't mean she was giving up. As the month ended, I went for a morning walk through my neighborhood.

"How ya doing?" she asked me.

I glanced around, but she was just a voice this morning. I tried not answering her, to see if she would go away.

"My, you're looking handsome on this fine day!" she punted.

This was such a shock, so rare, that I blurted, "I'm a year older. I can't decide if that's a good thing or a bad thing."

"You can't do anything about it, so suck it up."

I was near the trolley tracks, and the lights began flashing. Alarms rang, and the barriers came down to block the street. I looked to see where the trolley was, because I was about to walk over the tracks, but Heather blurted out:

"I've got this one! Don't bother looking, you're fine. You're the Indestructible Man."

I walked straight for the tracks, feeling invulnerable, and then the trolley blasted past not three feet in front of me.

And it all seemed good: Heather; trolley; Nina hit by a truck; not paying attention to traffic; the end of all good things. It was all okay. I was fine.

The trolley blasted past, and after it was gone I carried on with my walk. Heather did not comment, and as wild as it seems to say this, I didn't really connect this incident with her or my illness again for months.

August: brain tumor

In early August I paid off a nagging debt that I had incurred early on in my illness, back in 2007 or so. Now I intended to put some money into savings for a few months and beef up my available cash.

Unfortunately, I wasn't able to follow through on this plan, because I had spent so much money on manic spending sprees. So instead of saving some cash, I applied hundreds of dollars to manic-debt reduction. In addition to constant worry about my illness, I felt anxiety pretty much all the time, anxiety about finances and whether I was going to run off one afternoon and buy a used car or some other disaster.

Early in August I went hiking on Mount Woodson with my friend Steve. It was a hot day, and we carried plenty of water. I had done this hike before, and so this time we came in from a direction I had not explored. The trail wound its way up the mountain, the sun was plenty warm, and the route was not too full of other hikers. We took on the gentle inclines at the beginning parts of the trail, and then we hit the rough part. Here there was a series of upward inclines where the trail crews had put rows of rocks across the way, to keep the trail from washing out during winter rains. So, hikers had to constantly lift their feet up and over these rows of rocks, for a distance of about a mile.

"These are the Staircases of Doom," Steve said, half in jest and half in aggravation.

"Yeah," I said. "Feel the burn."

We laughed and climbed over the next dozen rows of rocks, and by the time we got to the top of the mountain our calves were on fire.

"I'm tired," Steve said. "Bet we really feel this, come tomorrow morning."

"Those staircases tired me out, too," I said.

"Not me," Heather said. "I'm fine. You're a pansy. Try Everest; now *that* is a mountain."

I ignored this, and she didn't push it. Steve and I went to the famous Potato Chip Rock, but there were tons of hikers there, and we decided not to take our picture on top of the rock. Potato Chip Rock is a boulder which has broken apart, and one of the pieces juts out like a ledge, maybe eight or ten feet long. Hikers climb up the rock and scoot out to the end, and their friends take their pictures. I've never heard of anyone falling off the ledge, but I suppose it could happen, say, if the hiker was drunk.

The views from the top of the mountain were great; my favorite feature of the land below was an orchard of trees with dark green leaves. Oranges? Grapefruit? Avocadoes? Who knew?

Our trip down was of course much easier than the trip up, though we still sweated a good deal. On the Staircases of Doom I saw a rattlesnake coiled up on a rock, and I stopped moving. It took only a few moments before I blinked the sweat out of my eyes, and when I opened them again, there was no snake. I am pretty sure that was a hallucination, and on that theory, I didn't mention it to Steve.

Eventually we came off the mountain and went to a small convenience store, where we got cold drinks.

"Now *that* hits the spot," he said, and I nodded as I chugged a bottle of lemonade.

For the next few days I was pretty sore in the legs, but the hike had been about nine miles, in summer heat, and we did great. I felt pleased to be out exercising and staying in touch with nature.

In the mornings the air was cool, and every day, seven days a week, I got up before sunrise and read a few pages out of whatever book I was interested in at the moment. Then I took my daily walk. There was little traffic on the streets at this time of day, and the homeless were all asleep on the sidewalk.

One morning I walked down the street on the way to the café, and I saw a homeless man crouched against the wall of a building. He had no shirt and was deeply tanned, and his pants were full of holes and were filthy. His hair was an unkempt mess, and his tennis shoes were ripped up and caked with crud.

I didn't want to look too long at him, because inevitably when you do that with homeless people, they will hit you up for money. I wasn't in the mood for this, so I looked away. Then I felt vaguely bad for ignoring him, and I looked back. No one was there. Twenty feet away lay another sleeping homeless man, but the guy I had seen was merely a hallucination.

These visual symptoms started happening more frequently. Out on the streets I saw homeless people; in my room I saw maggots, beetles, cockroaches, and bugs I couldn't identify. This happened every few days and sometimes twice a day.

About ten days into the month I went on my morning walk and went past a large building that had once been a movie theater, but it had gone out of business. Half a dozen homeless people sat on the sidewalk, in various states of undress, and three police officers stood a few yards away. No one was yelling or making threats, but the scene seemed filled with tension. Fearing that this was the start of a class war that would draw me in and get me killed, I looked away and continued to walk.

Then, wondering how this situation with cops and homeless would play out, I glanced back again. There was one cop and one homeless person, and it looked like the cop was laughing at something the homeless person had said. The cop glanced up at me, and I waved, just to be friendly. A few seconds later I walked behind the building and out of sight.

I went and saw my psychiatrist and told her about these

hallucinations and the fact that they were becoming more frequent.

"Let's switch medicines," she said. "If your current anti-psychotic isn't working, there are others we can try. They have side effects..." She named half a dozen known side effects for the drug she put me on.

"I'll stay tuned," I promised, and that was all she could do.

Around mid-month my mother called, while I was in my room, after hauling a few bags of groceries home. She and I talked for a minute, just catching up, and then my mother said, "We had an emergency about a week ago. Your father woke up partially paralyzed, and he couldn't speak. I called 9-1-1, and they sent an ambulance and took him to the local hospital, and *they* sent him to a better-equipped hospital in Lexington.

"To make a long story short, he had a brain tumor. The doctors took it out, and he's no longer paralyzed, but his speech is slurred, and he can barely walk. He's resting now, so I'm not going to ask him to come to the phone, but we need everyone to say a prayer."

"He's not taking care of himself," said Heather. "Too much beer, and not enough exercise—"

Knock it off, I snapped at her, in my thoughts.

"Surly little bitch," she said to me.

"I hope he can overcome this," I said, but the words sounded feeble to me.

"His regular doctor said it will take months of physical therapy to get him walking again. We thought it was bad before, his having to use a walker to get around, but we got a real wake-up call this time. I took it for granted, when he didn't get worse for a while, that maybe he had beat it. No one knows but God, and He isn't telling. I'll let you know how he's doing, as we go along."

We talked a few minutes more, about what I was up to, and then she had other people to call, and she hung up. I closed my cell phone and put it away. My father was virtually confined to bed and the couch, he had months of physical therapy in front of him, and there was always the chance that the cancer would come back. It could grow another tumor in his brain, or it could attack other vital organs. I wondered if my dad was entering his final year of life.

Over the space of a few days I realized my situation and his were similar. I too had been scanned, back in late 2009 or early 2010. My primary care doctor at the time found no tumors or abnormalities in my brain. But *something* was wrong in there, and if it wasn't a tumor, it was bad chemicals or misfiring neurons giving me trouble.

So my dad and I were both suffering ill health due to problems in our brains, and it was a toss-up to see who would lose the most, the fastest: him, or me?

I worried about the prospect that my father would grow worse instead of getting better, and I sent emails to friends telling them about this situation. My friends said kind words, and I received "support" from my delusions, too: every two or three days, as I thought about my dad's long fight with cancer, someone jostled glass bottles or dropped them on the sidewalk, and I knew that this meant all my worries about my dad's brain tumor would be "recycled" and would repeat themselves.

As I realized this and braced myself for my father's continued battles, a big dog somewhere on the sidewalk outside gave a loud bark. In the architecture of my illness, my dad was *owned* by one of the biggest dogs of all, death, and he was going to have to really fight to get out of the clutches of the bone man.

It's a sobering thought, that your one and only dad might die soon, and I was down-hearted for about a week as I thought it over. For some reason Heather didn't say much about this, and in fact, she hardly showed up at all.

Now, I was in the habit of buying a couple bottles of wine a week, and drinking a glass or two every day. I got into this habit years ago, when there was a series of media reports claiming that a glass of red wine a day was good for your heart. So I figured that in addition to daily walks and a couple of hikes a month, I would keep my heart healthy by drinking red wine.

But as I thought over my dad's sickness, I wondered if that wine really was good for my health. The booze was pricey, and I found I didn't want to keep this habit up.

So I stopped drinking wine; I drained my last glass and then started drinking fruit juice instead. Apple juice, cranberry juice, vegetable juice, and so on, favoring whatever was on sale.

The effect was almost immediate: I *felt* physically better and healthier. I could drink a couple full glasses a day for the same price as a single half glass of wine. I told my friends about this change, and they cheered me on.

"Now try to go vegetarian," my friend Daniel told me.

"That's too much," I said. "I still like meat, especially seafood."

"It's really healthy to give up red meat," he declared.

My friend Steve said, "My mother died of dementia-related symptoms. It was horrible to watch her slowly lose herself, and I have changed my diet so I can avoid what happened to her. Every day I eat blueberries, because they're supposed to be good for my brain. As for you, though, this is a good step forward. Eat right, drink healthy, and exercise regularly. Maybe we'll be in the same old age home, living 'til we're ninety-nine!"

Around mid-month I had a nasty little run-in with the past. I went for a routine check-up with my primary care doctor, and I mentioned a lump in my scrotum. He checked it out and sent me for an ultrasound scan. The scan came back negative: the lump was not cancer or problematic. It was just a side effect of the vasectomy I had, in 2007.

In my first memoir I discussed at some length my experiences in Egypt in 2007, but there was one that I did not share in *Randal, Randal, Burning Bright*. It has to do with my gonads, and here it is:

Sometime in May or June the days started warming up, and I could tell that Cairo, the capital city of Egypt and the largest city in the Middle East, was going to be hot soon. I stayed in cheap hotels and ate in noodle shops, and I sat in cafes every day smoking the hookah pipes and reading books of Arab folktales. At this point in my journey I had money, but I knew it was going to run out in a couple weeks, and my friends and family weren't inclined to fly me back to the States.

Heather hounded me day after day and sounded like this: "You are suffering bad health. You seem to be mentally ill. When are you going to take care of yourself?" She inserted a picture in my mind, a picture of a carved stone relief of the ancient Egyptian god Min. This god had one outstanding feature: his erect penis stood up and stuck out prominently.

She said, "You're sick in the head. Your dick is sick, too. You need to go to the hospital."

I could only imagine the horrors of an Egyptian hospital, and for days I fought her comments. She fought back:

"If you don't get help you'll get worse, and the Egyptians will lock you up in the nut house. You need to show you're willing to work with the doctors to get you back to health."

With these comments came a fierce urge to go to the hospital. I asked an Egyptian at the front desk of the hotel I was staying in at this point, and he told me the name of the biggest, best hospital in Cairo. It was just a short taxi ride away, and, pushed by Heather, I went at once.

The taxi driver stopped in front of the hospital, and I paid him. He left, and I stood there for a while, wondering what was going to happen to me.

"Look around your feet," Heather said. "See that piece of glass? Pick it up."

I saw the shattered bottle and said, "Why?"

"I have figured out what is wrong with you. You have

testosterone poisoning. You need to pick up that piece of glass and cut your balls off with it. Sooner, the better."

The fragment of glass was clear, and I figured it would do the job she had suggested.

"I'm not going to do that," I said feebly. I was so worried about running out of money that I could hardly fight with her. "There's nothing wrong with my nuts."

"I'm telling you," she purred, "That you need to stop that flow of bad chemicals to your brain. Now do it."

We fought for a good five minutes, back and forth. Sometimes she had the upper hand, and I reached for the glass fragment, and sometimes I got ahead, and I tried to ignore her. At last I walked away from the glass.

Heather screamed: "You no-good, worthless son-of-a-bitch! You complain all the time about me and the other voices, you whine constantly about your pain and your misery, but now you won't put it to an end?! There's nothing wrong with your brain except an excess of nut juice. I'll be on you tomorrow, and the next day, and the next, and God as my witness, you'll slice those little raisins right off."

I knew she could do this. She could get me to go places I didn't want to go, and she could get me to say things she wanted me to say, and I was sure she could get me to castrate myself, if she worked on me long enough.

"I'll get a vasectomy," I blurted. "That much I'll do."

"Yaay!" she howled gleefully.

I felt very strange about this, but I went into the hospital and told them I wanted a vasectomy. It took a few tries, until they found me a doctor who spoke English, and he sent me to a private clinic. There I had the operation. It cost six hundred dollars, and the doctor did it in about an hour.

Heather giggled. "Next time I'll have you cut your *head* off!"

Of course having this operation didn't cure my mental illness, or even reduce the symptoms. The voices were quiet for a few days, and I walked very carefully around Cairo with my genitals in a large cotton bandage. I was very sore, and I wondered what would have happened if I had not forged this compromise with Heather. Would I really have cut my testicles off? It didn't matter, did it? What mattered is that she *might* have been able to get me to do it, and I had to respond to that threat.

Back in the present day, August 2016, I remembered this experience in Cairo, and I was glad my primary care doctor found nothing wrong with me. As I get older, I am more concerned about my health, and with Heather and the minor voices in my head, there are enough threats to my well-being to make me concerned much of the time. It seemed to me that Heather had been stronger then, or maybe it was just that the battlefield had become more subtle since my time in Cairo.

I exited the hospital after seeing my primary care doctor, and Heather appeared, behind me. I turned around to see her, and she moved out of sight. Or became invisible. At any rate, I felt her presence but couldn't see her.

"You never had a vasectomy," she said. "It was fake."

I walked to the bus stop in front of the VA hospital and sat down on a chair; there were several other people there, waiting for the bus.

So my primary care doctor found the same lump I did, and he's just making up stories about vasectomies? Why would that be?

Her voice seemed right over my head, but I didn't lean back to see her. "Once you release this material, you'll sell a zillion books. Hearing voices, Chinese out of Tibet, billion dollars, sitting there with your pants down for an hour while the Egyptian doctor slashed up your nuts."

My nuts swelled up and stayed that way for a week. Blood all over the place. There were real wounds.

"All fake," she said. "You're in the program. 9/11 was fake, all these unarmed black men the police are supposedly killing are fake, your vasectomy was fake… There's a ton of this stuff. It would take me an hour to rip apart what you 'know' about the last ten years that never happened, or was actually about you. You're *supposed* to come to LA, find me, and help me build my career while we raise our three kids. Anything that gets in the way of that, well…not pretty."

This made me dizzy, and I stopped talking with her. The bus arrived, and when I got home I dropped my shorts and looked at my scrotum: two small scars. But she had gotten to me, and I could no longer tell if I had really had my nuts cut or if this was the latest crime against me by a global conspiracy.

It could have been my decision to drink fruit juice instead of wine, but in any event I did a lot of hiking in August. Late in the month I hiked Tecolote Canyon with my friend Daniel. That's about an eight mile trail. Every morning I walked a mile and a half, and I took several trips up to Balboa Park and hiked Trail #5 and Trail #13. By the end of the month I had put about 75 miles under my feet, and I went into September feeling pretty good.

Down Cycle

September: thoughts from friends

September didn't start off bad. My symptoms were moderate, and maybe that was due to the change in medications? Also, I was walking and hiking frequently, and that exercise might have had something to do with feeling good. We were in an El Nino year, weather-wise, and the daily temperatures were notably cooler than usual. In fact, it was downright nice out. I could almost believe that my illness was going to get better.

In the spirit of starting the month off right, I took a walk along the harbor. The day was pleasantly warm, and there was a gentle breeze off the water. I just walked, with no real idea where to go, and in no time I passed by the airport and kept going. Finally I reached a little grassy park, with some open structures that looked vaguely like shrines. There were plaques here and there, and I read those: the place was named Cancer Survivors Park. Instantly I thought of my dad. Some of the words were in tribute to those who had fought their cancer and won, and some of them honored those who had fought and died. I didn't know which of these my father was destined for.

I walked around the park and read everything, and I said a little prayer that my dad would get his health back and have twenty more excellent years yet.

About a week after this, I re-read an article that had really shaken me, in the news media. It was a grim piece. At the time the article was written, July of 2016, more than 500 Americans had been killed by the police for that year. Of those, about one in four were mentally ill. The mainstream media makes a big show of keeping count of unarmed black men who are killed by police each year, and only recently have journalists and advocacy groups started tallying the death toll among the mentally ill.

I had read the story before, but I still didn't know what to make of it. The article gave some specific examples of mentally ill people who were killed, and the reporter who wrote it talked with the families of the slain people and the police themselves, trying to figure out how hundreds of mentally ill people die at the hands of police officers each year.

From the police viewpoint, these situations boiled down to two factors: mentally ill people act weird or unpredictably, and they often refuse to obey instructions from the police.

From time to time I had seen articles that reported specific mentally ill individuals who had been killed by the police, but *two hundred and fifty a year?* What the hell was *that* all about? I wondered about it, but I had my own mental illness to keep me busy, and it didn't occur to me at this juncture to look up any more articles of this type. However, it was the first spark of an idea: *how deep did this go?* Over a hundred mentally ill people killed by police so far in 2016, and who knew how many for previous years? It gave me chills to think of this. Then I remembered the article I had read before, that mentally ill people were sixteen times more likely to be killed by the police than healthy people.

I had no idea what to do with this information, but it sure as hell seemed clear that I needed to stay far away from the cops. They were looking for mentally ill people to kill, and Heather was looking to sic them on me. One two combo punch, and that would be the end of me.

For a few weeks I had exchanged emails with a lady friend who is a lawyer, as we discussed our ideas about God. She said her piece, and then I said, "I suppose God may be good, but ask the Jews in Auschwitz about how God is merciful and compassionate, and see what they say."

"I'm not comfortable thinking that way," she said. "You have to accentuate the positive."

"What would have happened if the Jews had armed themselves

against the Nazi who came to send them to the concentration camps? There are evil people in this world, and they will kill you if you don't fight back. In the end, it comes down to who is willing to shoot whom," I said, and that got me thinking about the cops merrily blowing away every mentally ill person they came across.

A few days went by, and I hiked Cowles Mountain on my own. It was a short jaunt, just three miles round trip, and the weather was pleasant. At the top I stared at the distant mountains to the east and daydreamed a huge dragon curled up on its treasure pile on top El Cajon Mountain. This small exercise of imagination felt good, and physically I felt good, too, as I hiked back down Cowles and crossed the street to a Mexican eatery to have a meal.

As I ate the burrito, my thoughts went back to, "Who was willing to shoot whom?" How would history have been different if a million Jewish people had armed themselves and gone after the Nazis? Somehow, when the guns come out, it's always the wrong people who are armed. The brutes, the Nazis, the criminals. And the first thing they do is pass laws stating that anyone who dares defend themselves is the *real* criminal.

These thoughts made me want a gun. Years and years ago, all the way back in 2008, I had been a proud gun owner. I never used my pistol for anything and just carried it around in the trunk of my car. Then the cops in Las Vegas, Nevada seized the weapon during a search of my car, and that ended my ability to defend myself. Now, I guessed, I was at the mercy of whoever wanted to shoot me first. This was a sobering, even sickening idea, and I wondered what it would take to get my gun back from the LVPD. But no, they had probably held onto it for a few months, and once I didn't go get it, they had sold it at auction.

A few days passed, and the paranoid thoughts about guns and cops and murdered mentally ill people continued. Heather didn't pipe up, but my illness began to escalate. It was clear that the police were not merely willing to shoot the mentally ill, they purposely escalated these encounters until the mentally ill person charged them, and then the cops blew them away. This was not 'law enforcement:' it was 'blood sport.' Cops with guns on one side, broken down sicklings on the other side. Let the games begin!

These bursts of paranoia continued, and I became certain that the police were going to kill me, or put me in jail, or send me to the loony bin. Heather stayed gone much of the time, which made me think she was setting up for a big attack of some sort. I became worried all the time and thought I could hear people plotting against me at the café, sending me their hostile thoughts just to show they could.

I went hiking with Daniel and his wife and daughter at Los Penasquitos Canyon Preserve. The weather was delightful; we walked three miles on the trail and arrived at a small waterfall where we sat down on some rocks and ate snacks. Daniel and his daughter took off their shoes and splashed around in the pool under the waterfall. A dozen adults also sat on the rocks, and several little kids walked around in the water near my friends.

Daniel's wife and I sat and talked. For a few minutes we spoke about the hike, and how mild today's weather was compared to the same time last year.

Then she looked me right in the eyes. She is Japanese-American, and English is her second language. "Help me understand," she said.

"About what?" I responded.

"About this illness you have. This mental illness. Some woman is your make-believe girlfriend? That is what Daniel told me. What does she say to you? And, she is only in your mind?"

"Yes. Sometimes I see her, like a ghost, or an image, but most of the time she is just a voice in my head. She says things like, 'Randal, you're so stupid,' and 'Come to Los Angeles with me, and let's have kids!' She goes on like that for hours, day after day."

"Why?" she asked. "Where did this voice come from?"

"I don't know why she shows up, or where she came from. She's been in my head for years."

"And the medicine doesn't get rid of her?"

"It helps so she can't make as much noise; it quiets her down."

"There are other voices, too?" she asked me.

"Yes, sometimes just one or two and sometimes half a dozen. But they're not really personalities, like Heather. They're just noisy."

"How many years have you been taking these medicines, and they don't work?"

"Some of them work. The lithium seems to have stabilized my moods, so I'm not manic all the time. The anti-psychotic is making Heather a little quieter." I had told most of this to Daniel over the years, in dribs and drabs, but it looked like he had only passed a little of that on to his wife.

"But, with the medicine, shouldn't this imaginary person go away? Why is she coming around? Why can't the medicine make her be quiet? How long ago did you get sick?"

"It's been over ten years," I said, and she looked amazed. "At least I have housing now, and I'm not living on the streets. My psychiatrist does everything she can do, and things get a little better. She can't work miracles; she can only try this and try that and see what helps."

"How did you get sick to start with?"

"No one knows."

"This is no good!" she blurted. "You don't have cancer or something else that's real. How many psychiatrists have tried to make you better?"

"Five or six."

"And they can't stop this Heather person? Nothing works?"

"I had a brain scan a few years ago, and there was no tumor or damage to my brain. My illness may be a chemical imbalance in my brain, or it may be a problem with my mind and not my brain at all."

She nodded vigorously. "I have been telling our daughter about your situation. I told her you are sick, and she wanted to know what was wrong with you. But that made me realize that *I* don't really understand it, so how could I explain to her?"

"It's complicated," I started, and she quickly cut me off.

"It's easy to see what is going on," she said forcefully. "Let me tell you what I see."

"Okay," I said. "Like what?"

"You're not mentally ill," she said with the same forcefulness. "Here's what's happening to you: you sit in your little room, day after day, and read books about mentally ill people. You read the articles online, and those are all negative: mentally ill people are killers! Mentally ill people are dangerous! And other people say, 'the mentally ill people need help, and housing, and psychiatrists! You told me once that some of your friends are mentally ill, and you talk with them all the time."

"It's important to find out about my condition," I said. "If you were sick, wouldn't you read up on it?"

"Yes, I would, but if I had an illness that went on for ten years, I would get a different doctor! You know what I think?"

"Hit me," I said.

"You make yourself sick by paying so much attention to mental illness."

"If I didn't pay so much attention to my illness, I'd probably be dead by now."

"Think about it," she said, in an exasperated tone of voice. "Ten years?"

Then Daniel and their daughter came out of the stream, and we hiked the three miles back to the parking lot.

On the trip back to my room, Daniel, who was driving, suddenly said, "You never talk about looking for work, Randal. But you do your hobbies every day. How many hours a day is that? Reading, and writing, and daily exercise? Isn't that a kind of work?"

Now *he* was after me, and I didn't know what to make of it.

"If you're working, you make money," I said. "That's the difference between a hobby and a job."

"Don't you make money from your writing? Don't you put your books up for sale?"

"Yes, and I make about fifty bucks a year from royalties."

"That's a lot of money," said my goddaughter, who was seven years old.

"Ha ha, that won't pay rent for even one month," I said to her.

"You should try it," said Daniel's wife. "You should put your hobbies aside and get a job. Not full-time, I know you can't do that…"

"If you can read and write for four hours a day, you can do a half-time job four hours a day," Daniel said. "Find something simple you can do, like sit in a booth in a parking garage and punch people's tickets. Something like that, that is low-stress."

"I have a masters degree," I said sharply. "I'm not going to accept eight bucks an hour punching tickets."

"Well, find *something* for work," said Daniel's wife. "You're just taking money away from tax payers like us, so you can make yourself feel bad by reading too many media stories about mental illness. Like I said before."

"Really, you should at least *try*," Daniel said.

Then they dropped me off at home.

All these comments slammed into my mind like a bull in a china shop. When should I expect to get better? *Was* I feeding my own illness? I knew I wasn't making myself sick, like my friend's wife suggested, but her comment that I hadn't gotten well in ten years put my situation in stark relief.

What about getting a job? No way could I manage full time work, and I couldn't do anything that was very stressful. What did that leave? In the old days, before mental illness destroyed my life, I had been a web developer. I did some web design work, and I laid out information architecture for web sites under development, and I did lightweight programming like HTML and CSS and a little Javascripting. I didn't make tons of money, but I had a tidy little life.

I hadn't worked in over ten years, and my skills were no longer up-to-date. What kind of job could I reasonably look for?

As the month of September wound down into its final week, a new set of questions occurred to me, like: why the hell were my friends so insistent I look for a job, all of a sudden? Because their daughter asked what kind of sickness I had, and that got them asking questions of their own?

Ten years without getting better? But no, I was a little improved. Certainly I was better off than when I was living in a cement drainage culvert in the Santa Fe winter, all those years ago. The medicines, and the CBSST techniques, had taken some of the edge off the symptoms.

I walked to the café with a book to read and bought a coffee.

"There's nothing wrong with you," Heather said. "You just need some great sex, and a couple kids to take care of."

You should just leave, I thought, with a distinct lack of enthusiasm. There were only a few people in the café, and I sat down at a table and tried to ignore her. I felt a keen sense of irony in that the voices in my head were the ones telling me I wasn't mentally ill.

"I've been thinking," Heather said, and then I could see her, out of the corner of my eye, sitting at another nearby table. She wore a heavy blouse and jeans, and as she talked she curled up one hand and held it under her chin. She looked like that famous statue, "The Thinker."

Thinking about what?

"You take all these stupid walks and hikes all over the place. You look up stupid flowers and birds, in nature books. Maybe you should do that for your job. Be a park ranger. There are so many stupid parks in San Diego County that the rangers can put you out of the way in a park no one ever goes to. How's that?"

Park rangers carry guns, I said. *Can you imagine how things would go if I started hallucinating insects all over the place, and I took out my pistol and shot every bug I saw? Yeah, that's a stroke of genius, Heather.*

"When you get your billion dollars, you'll find your new job, which is 'world-famous writer.' And husband. And father of three rug rats. It just gets better from there."

When does the Nobel Committee award the peace prize?

"You keep coming back to that. Who cares? You'll get it when they give it. Isn't the money more important?"

Recognition is more important.

"Then do something amazing."

According to what you said a few months ago, I already have done amazing things. When do I get my rewards?

"I'm not in charge of that," she said.

This made me very angry, and I finished reading the chapter in the book. I got up with my coffee and left the café. Heather followed me but stayed quiet as I went for a walk. For eight or ten blocks everything was all right, but as I got to a traffic intersection and stepped off the curb, Heather said,

"You can go! No problem! I'm got us covered."

So I trotted out into the intersection, and suddenly a driver slammed his horn and screeched to a stop just a few yards away. The noises made my heart lurch in my chest, and I became disoriented.

The angry driver kept slamming his horn, and I looked at the flow of traffic and ran across the street.

"God *damn* it, Heather!" I yelped, from the safety of the sidewalk. "You said you were looking!"

"I have us covered," she said. "You're asking a lot of stupid questions these last couple weeks. I've told you all you need to know about your illness. Good things will come your way. You have to be strong enough to *deserve* them."

"I think the Nobel winners are announced in October," I said.

"The prize committee announces the awards when it makes sense to do so," she said with anger.

"It's the FUCKING NOBEL PRIZE!" I barked, as a few cars went by.

Suddenly I knew the drivers of those cars were on their hands-free phones, calling the cops to report a man running into traffic and trying to commit suicide.

"It's not *suicide*," Heather said. "I'm just checking to see that you trust me more than you trust your own feeble instincts. You need people on your side. I'm taking care of you, dumb fuck."

Just to be sure the cops couldn't find me, I cut through a small park near the trolley tracks and went a different route than I usually followed. In fifteen minutes I arrived home; no cops tried to kill me.

For the rest of the month I went walking every morning, and sometimes in the afternoon. The weather was superb, cool and usually with a fresh breeze off the ocean. San Diego had really had a great summer, and I was pleased at all the exercise I had chalked up.

My mother called and told me, "Your dad went in for treatment. The doctor called this a 'gamma knife; it's radiation straight into his brain. The doctors haven't found any sign of cancer, but one of them told me that when they remove a tumor, there are sometimes bits of cancer left behind. So this treatment is to kill those."

"How did it go?" I asked, feeling sick as I empathized with my father's ill health. "How is he doing?"

"He feels awful, but he said it's better to be safe than sorry. What can we do? We have to fight with everything we've got."

"Yes," I agreed.

"This brings it home, you know?" she said. "We really could lose him."

"I wish I could help," I said.

"I'll call you if anything changes. I hope this gamma knife got the last of it, but it seems like there's always another treatment to try. I wish the drugs and the radiation were more effective. He shouldn't by utterly miserable for years on end. That is crazy."

"How are you doing?" I asked her.

"I'm okay. I feel like your dad's struggle is my struggle, and it wears me out. It's tiring to wonder every day what is going to happen next."

"Sometimes I wish I had super-powers," I said.

"It's in God's hands now, whichever way it goes. I have to get back to him, he needs me. Take care of yourself."

"You, too," I said, and I cut the connection.

It was clear that if my dad's health was up to God, he was screwed. Auschwitz, Treblinka, Dachau, and on and on. God very clearly played favorites, or He had abdicated all responsibility for the human race and allowed monsters like the Nazis to do whatever they want. Free will to the max, and Devil take the hindmost.

So, how did my dad's situation stack up? Cut out the skin cancer, cut out the infected lymph nodes nearest the skin cancer, round after round of chemo, brain tumor, gamma knife, and of course lots of prayers. No wonder he and my mother were tired all the time.

At the end of September I sat down and tallied up all the hikes and walks, and as near as I could estimate, I had put ninety miles on my hiking shoes in that one month. After each individual walk I felt good, but my feet were sore pretty much all the time, and there were these little needles in my soles that hurt when I tried to sleep.

Outside my window, a big dog let out a single, aggressive bark. I took it that either Heather or the cops were going to come down on me like a ton of bricks.

October: what scares you

October is of course Halloween month, and I checked a book of ghost stories out of the library and read them in the mornings, before the sun rose each day. The stories were oldies, from the eighteenth and nineteenth centuries, and they were fun to read.

But my mind was not clear. My friends slamming on me to get a job really haunted me. Ghosts and devils and evil spirits were just an amusement, and as my father faced attack after attack from cancer, angels and good spirits seemed distant or just a dream we foster for children, to keep the night terrors away.

Daniel and I hiked Sycamore Canyon, an eight mile route on a warm day. There were some good hills, and the walk along the ridgetops was a great time. But my feet hurt, like pins and needles sticking into my soles, and by the time we hiked the full circuit and back to his car, I could hardly walk. He drove me home.

The next day I tried to take my normal daily walk, but my feet hurt so bad I couldn't do it. Even a mile and a half was too much, and I had to quit and return to my room. I looked up bone spurs, and vascular conditions, but these didn't seem to fit the bill for what I was experiencing. Somewhere along the way I found information on plantar fasciitis, and that sounded right. An article I read online said you have to get off your feet—no long walks, no hiking—and stay off them for a couple of months.

This set the stage for a miserable October. I stopped walking except by necessity—to the grocery store and so forth, and I cancelled all my hikes for the rest of the year. Every morning I went to the café, and then I just…went home. It was like my legs were pleading with me to try a walk, just a short walk, give it a whirl, huh? But I had read articles that said flat-out, if you walk on injured feet, the injury will become worse and might require surgery to repair.

I didn't get out and around the neighborhood, and I didn't chat with the dog walkers anymore, and I even missed the homeless people I thought were all out to get me. The cops stayed in their police station or patrolled somewhere away from me, and when I mentioned my aching feet to my friends, Steve said it sounded like plantar fasciitis, and he'd had it too.

"Give it a few weeks to clear up on its own, and if it doesn't, get to the doctor and let him take a look at it," he said. "It could be something serious. With my plantar, my doctor gave me a pair of shoe inserts, and that did the trick. If I over-exert, the plantar starts hurting again, but that hasn't happened in years."

On top of foot pain, my mania kicked into high gear. I kept spending too much money and could barely keep up with my credit card payments. Every excess purchase I made seemed "reasonable" from the point of view of my manic brain. Didn't I deserve goodies for putting up with Heather and plantar and not being able to take walks? And it seemed something was always breaking down or falling apart and needed to be replaced. I thought maybe it would be fun to take a trip up to San Francisco for a few days and visit some old friends up there. I hadn't taken a vacation in 2016, and wasn't I due some enjoyment?

As I contemplated the expenses involved in travel, Heather said,

"You should just move to San Francisco. You're always complaining that The City has more cultural events, that Muir Woods is nearby, that wine country is just a short drive away…all that crap."

"I was thinking of moving to Santa Fe," I said, "But I haven't been able to save any money."

"And now you want to do what, go deep into debt for travel you can't afford? You're not only not learning from your experiences, you're getting stupider as you go. Don't *visit* there; move there."

Something about her criticism brought this home to me. I wanted to pay off my credit cards, and instead I was running them up to the max.

What the hell was I going to do, incur another eight hundred dollar debt in spur-of-the-moment travel?

Of course, there's never a fire of bad news burning so hot that someone can't dump some gasoline on it. Namely, I called my parents and actually got my dad on the line.

"How's it going?" I asked him.

He sounded enervated as he returned, "Kind of tired. It's not so bad when I rest, but it kills me to do anything."

"Are you going to be able to go deer hunting this year?" I asked him. "You could sit in your stand and blast 'em as they come past."

"No, I'm not going to have strength for that," he said in a weak voice.

"A holiday season of rest," I offered.

"You know, those doctors, they tell you the treatments are going to wear you down. But Holy Moly, they really kick my butt!" His voice became a little stronger, and I laughed along with him.

"It's one damned thing after the next," he said, his voice getting weak again. "My doctor here, he says this brain tumor may come back. I don't know. I don't know about more fights with cancer. Each time I go a couple rounds with it, I get more tired than the last time. Can't I beat this for once and for all?"

"I feel the same way about my disorder," I said. "Every time I go into an up cycle, I say, 'Is that the last of it? Am I free?'"

"You've had that crap for a long time," he said.

"Ten years," I said. "I'm in another down cycle. Started last month, and now it's getting worse. I was hoping this would be a good holiday season, but all bets are off."

"You'd think with all those drugs the psychiatrists are having you take, that something would work."

"The lithium was doing a good job for months," I said. "Maybe it's time to crank up the dose."

"It's good talking to you, but I have to go. I can't talk for long. You going anywhere for Christmas?"

"Hadn't planned on it. Keep up the good fight, dad."

"You too. We're a pair of cripples. Somebody should shoot both of us and put us out of our misery."

I laughed, and he hung up the phone.

A few days after this I woke up with a sharp, clear idea in my mind. I was going to write a memoir in 2017, which is the book you hold here in your hands. I thought it would be interesting to follow up on my illness for a relatively short period and to show the differences in the symptoms as they evolved over time. Most of all, I decided, I would discuss the details of my symptoms. Many people who write mental illness memoirs gloss the symptoms in favor of staying focused on how disruptive the illness is to the relationships of the mentally ill person. I wanted to give symptoms front and center. All I needed to do was decide how to approach the writing of this second memoir, and what books I needed to read, for research.

It would not be appropriate to mention the spooks and witches of Halloween without also bringing up scary people who were in the news. The presidential election was coming up in just a few weeks, and the media was going nuts to provide as much idiotic, cheap-thrill-seeking, confrontational sound bites featuring this candidate or that one. Both major parties declared theirs to be the best candidate for America, and of course the candidates from the other party were going to destroy the country.

For some reason this foo-foo-rah seemed unusually ugly this year, especially on social media where there are apparently no limits placed on what partisans of all stripes can say. My main grievance was, how did two geriatric candidates come to represent the best choice for president of the country? Did anyone expect either Hillary Clinton or Donald Trump to survive their term? Was this the start of a new trend of aged presidents seeking office?

The social media vitriol unleashed on both candidates unnerved me, and I experienced strong paranoia as I feared someone would shoot both candidates. Personal attacks went on and on, and political sharp-shooters from both parties seemed ready to spill blood.

After a week when it seemed everyone on social media was proclaiming Donald Trump to be a Nazi and Hillary Clinton to be a crook, Heather popped in. There was no visual hallucination this time, just her rather wary-sounding voice:

"The cops are going to kill Donald Trump, and guess who's going to be framed for it?"

My paranoia spiked high and sharp, and I could just picture a couple of bullet-head cops dragging me off to somewhere out of the way, where they'd kill me and say I had attacked *them* in a fit of mental illness. Similar paranoid scenes flashed through my mind in seconds, and they brought with them great fear, that my life really was going to be over soon.

"Have you been checking out these attack ads?" she asked. "They're really building up to this election, aren't they? Or should I say, this assassination?"

"How can I get them to stop?" I asked her. "How can I get the cops to leave me alone?"

"I think you know the answer to that one," she said.

But I didn't know what she meant, and I didn't know how to get out of this illness.

Over the next week my mania continued to blast, especially at night. The rush of too much energy would push-push-push me all afternoon and into the evening, and I woke up frequently and couldn't get back to sleep. At the same time paranoia and fear rolled through me, and every time I saw a police car I felt freaked-out and in the cross hairs.

Probably because of all the bad brain chemicals, and all the symptoms, and the side effects of my medicines, I had a hallucination so vivid it was more like a vision. I had eaten dinner and sat in front of my computer, and there was a bright light off to my right, in front of the refrigerator. I looked over there, and lo and behold, there was a full-sized angel, standing in a doorway made of light. I could only make out its outline, due to the brilliance of the light. The angel was dressed in a simple monk's robe, also white, and it reached out and beckoned me to enter the doorway.

My mouth went dry, and I croaked, "No, thanks."

The angel and the doorway and the light disappeared, and I sat there with my hands shaking, because what the hell had that been all about? Near-death experience? Touch of the afterlife? An answer to my question to Heather, about how do I get out of this mess?

Heather didn't show up to give her opinion, and I decided the angel was a response to stress over my father's health, and my own fragile mental state. And on and on the attack ads played on social media, and I soaked up the ugliness and the hate and struggled with the very real question of which candidate would be *less* likely to get us into a nuclear war with Asian powers.

I was diagnosed with schizoaffective disorder all the way back in 2008. Every once in a while I read a few online articles about this rare disorder, and I told all my friends about it and got their feedback. I've read memoirs about bipolar disorder, and memoirs about depression, and I decided I would start looking at more information about schizoaffective disorder.

I came across a lot of people talking about their symptoms in online forums, so I checked some of that out, and I read articles describing other people's course of treatment, as they looked for a miracle cure or at least medicine that wouldn't do them further harm. There were forums where you could weigh in with your experiences and your opinions, but I decided to stay out of this, because the people posting this information are not doctors or psychiatrists; their recommendations for what medicines to try are guesses based on how that drug performed for *them*.

My new anti-psychotic medicine seemed to be working in a limited way; Heather visited less frequently, which was heartening, but the mania kept going, day after day. A few days before the holiday I walked down the sidewalk and saw two hummingbirds. One was an Anna's hummingbird, and the other hummer looked like it was made of delicate plates of copper. The birds were definitely chirping back and forth to each other, and I had the idea that they were a mated pair. I knew there was a story there somewhere, but with my head as messed up as it was, it might be months before I could get it onto paper. Clearly they were hallucinations, but I couldn't figure out what they represented.

October ended with the Halloween holiday, which is always fun. I did the same thing I had done the previous year, which was to sit down on one of the window stools at my favorite café and watch all the costumed strollers go by. There were several young women dressed up in kitty-cat costumes, with whiskers drawn on their cheeks, and there were ghosts, and superheroes, and on and on.

At several points in the evening I saw strange events that I thought were some sort of precognition. Once I saw the image of a pickup truck for the public transportation organization, MTS, flash through my mind. I sat up, wondering what that was all about, and after a minute, an MTS truck went by.

A black-clad witch went by, and then I envisioned a government car coming near. Two minutes later, a black government sedan went by, its tinted windows hiding the people within.

Later that evening, I was thinking about the cops, and—you got it—a prowler went by. After everything else I was experiencing, a few psychic events seemed just like another freak at the circus.

November: light the fuse and run

I knew the cops were coming for me. They would shoot me outright or beat me half to death and then finish me off in prison; the details were vague, but the main thrust of the story was constant. November was a holiday month, but the only turkey was me.

"He gives a presidential pardon," Heather said blithely, a few days into the month.

The pain in my feet had reduced a bit, and so I was out on my daily walk and seeing if I could go back to exercising every day. I was also watching warily for police cars. Heather trotted alongside me, just out of the corner of my vision. "Pardon?" I croaked.

"President Obama. He gives a presidential pardon to a Thanksgiving turkey, every year. Every president does it. You should send an email to the White House, asking for a pardon." She sounded amused.

"I want my billion dollars," I blurted at her.

"It's right there in plain sight," she said. "Just figure out who has it, and approach them."

"If it's mine, why do I have to ask someone else for it?" I became angry, and I went on: "Or do the cops have it?"

"The cops have the bullet that's meant for your heart," she said flatly.

"God damn it, I haven't done anything! Why are the cops after me?"

"The cops and the mentally ill don't mix," she said. "You need to pay off the cops. Everyone does it. Why do you figure the politicians never get in trouble with the police? Payola." Then she disappeared, and I finished my walk.

At this point it would be wise to note that I had started reading Dante's *Inferno*, in an English translation. I found it hard going, because Dante referred to a lot of people and situations I was not familiar with. So the informative notes at the end of the chapters were invaluable.

What struck me most about the poem was the harsh treatment of pagans. Born before the time of Christ, they were barred from heaven and hell both and crowded around the entrance of hell, where they were sad shades with no lives and no future. Wasn't this the life of a mentally ill man in modern America? Sort of drifting along on SSDI, able to survive but not able to really live, spending a major portion of the day fighting symptoms, year after year.

On the 6th of November the San Diego Rescue Mission hosted a walk and candlelight vigil for the 115 homeless people who died in San Diego over the last year. That is, the homeless deaths the event organizers *knew about*. How many homeless people *really* died in a year, who knew? I joined about 100 other people, many wearing small metal crosses, and we started off by each of us picking up a pair of shoes marked with a name tag representing one homeless person who had died in the last year. I didn't get a pair of tennis shoes, or loafers, or what have you; I got a pair of hiking boots. The name on the tag was Marlon Williams, age 42. His death was somehow related to traffic or cars, but the tag did not elaborate. Marlon had been younger than me, just entering middle age. I wondered how long he had been homeless and if he was mentally ill, and I thought of his family and if the authorities had notified his loved ones of his death.

Carrying over a hundred pairs of such shoes, we walked to a nearby church, where the Christians among us sang a religious song to set the tone for the rest of the event. We walked to a second church and said a prayer, and then we walked to a government building where we held the vigil.

To me the best part of the event was when several people took turns reading off the 115 names. I didn't know any of those homeless people on the list, but I felt like I was with them in spirit. The whole walk and vigil took two hours, and I would participate again if the San Diego Rescue Mission holds this event once more, in the future.

Election day. I went to my polling place and did my duty. At the polling station were four or five Trump supporters with their "Make America Great Again" hats. I cast my vote and crept home to see how it turned out, and you know how that story goes....

Immediately there was a great series of shrieks from Hillary supporters, and the media was full of accusations of "stolen election," "hanging chads," and so forth. Some of my friends became extremely outspoken against Donald Trump, to the point where it became painful to read their posts on social media. Trump and Putin were shown as lovers in doctored photos, and it seemed that every little thing Donald Trump had ever said was recycled and held against him.

The most pernicious images, to me, were Trump with swastika armbands, or in full SS uniform, and so forth. The constant blast of anti-Trump posts really wore me out.

"Welcome to the death camps," a minor voice in my mind said, a few days after the election. "First Mexicans, then cripples, then liberals."

I didn't usually talk much with the minor voices. They came and spat their messages, and then they left. Sometimes they hung out for a few hours, but this one was apparently satisfied to light the fuse with incendiary speech, and then run.

I had read in the media, over the course of a few years, articles about lawmakers making comments against disabled people. Sometimes they talked about what a "burden" people with disabilities were, or a "drain on society." The president-elect had issued conflicting statements about disability, saying sometimes that he wasn't going to touch social security programs and other times that he was going to get rid of 'waste' and 'fraud,' to be defined later.

Spurred on by the political talk of cracking down on disabled people, I found a web site with forums for mentally ill people to talk about their conditions, their medicines, their health care situation, politics and disability, and so forth. For a couple weeks I stuck to the forum for schizoaffective disorder, and I read about the symptoms and the treatments that members of the community shared.

I ran across a set of articles about schizoaffective disorder, and I read them avidly. What stunned me about these articles was the writer's comment that he had been schizoaffective for almost twenty years, and during that time he experienced voices about once every three years. I read this, and then I went back and read it again. Once every *three years*. I, on the other hand, experienced voices and other psychotic symptoms about half a dozen times *a day*.

I had never really much explored other people's mental illness before; I assumed that everyone had symptoms that were roughly equivalent to my own. I thought *everyone* had their own private Heather, and *everyone* had a swarm of minor voices running games of buzzword bingo. Paranoia, attacks of terror, and cops gunning for them were part of the common experience of all people with schizoaffective disorder. As I've mentioned earlier, I have several friends who are bipolar, but that is a very different illness from schizoaffective disorder, and it's hard to compare symptoms.

So I was shocked to find that my supposition was not so. Some people on the forums had been diagnosed with the disorder, they got pills, and *viola*, the illness went away. Other people had been through the long road, like me: mental illness, job loss, homelessness and suicidal experiences, and eventual stabilization of symptoms, with the hope of recovery.

I didn't know what to say to the people who heard annoying voices once every six months. I wouldn't even call that mental illness, any more than I would call a mild scrape on your knee, a life-threatening injury. So I didn't post any messages; I just lurked and read other people's experiences and advice.

One thing I noticed was that very few people talked about getting better. They talked frequently about "managing symptoms," or "trying various anti-psychotic drugs," and some people claimed marijuana did wonders, or natural herbal remedies had relieved their symptoms. It occurred to me that probably the people who had gotten better quit posting in the forums and returned to their interrupted lives. That left the newbies, some of whom would get better, and the chronic cases, who no longer expected to recover.

At this point I still thought of myself as a lone sicko. But as I read these posts on the forums, I noticed how brave these people were. Some of them made jokes about their illness, and others talked about involuntary commitment to psych wards, or loss of their jobs due to psychotic episodes, and so forth. Many held out hope for finding a good combination of psych meds and talk therapy, and others found solace on the forums.

This range of symptoms and responses to symptoms got me thinking, and I really dug into the media to find out more about my long-term prognosis. Schizoaffective disorder is rare; less than one half of one percent of Americans suffer from this condition, but that meant something like a million of us have it. There should be a lot of good information out there.

Some internet booster once said that you can find any information you need on the internet, but for me this hasn't been true. You can find *common* knowledge on the net, and I think you can find damned near anything for sale, but finding information about rare mental illnesses is significantly harder. What I found, as I conducted my search, was that a lot of medical websites gave definitions of the disorder, and signs to look for that may indicate someone has the illness, and various medicines to treat it. Hospitals and treatment centers gave their pitch for why you should come to them for diagnosis and therapy, and so forth.

Finding out more about my illness seemed important, almost an obsession. I had suffered my illness for ten years, and I had found out a little about it but was mostly content to see my psychiatrist and take my meds on time. I had a good diet and ate healthy food, I usually got enough sleep, and yes, I exercised every day. It didn't take a genius to see that if these common-sense practices were really effective, I'd be cured by now.

So I dug around some more on the net, and then I found a study that followed schizoaffective sufferers for ten years. The outcome was not a surprise: about 25% of the SZA (schizoaffective) people recovered within two years of becoming ill, and 47% of SZA people got better within five years of becoming ill. Unfortunately, if you didn't get better within 10 years, your chances of recovery diminished sharply. So that meant that for me, I should quit expecting a recovery and start focusing on long-term symptom management.

I was not pleased at this conclusion, because American culture sells you the notion, that if you just do the right things you can have what you want. Consume the right products, follow the right routine, become friends with the right people, and so on, and success is all but guaranteed to be yours.

When the culture guarantees success through smart lifestyle choices, and the medical industry pushes "recovery" and holds up all these examples of famous mentally ill people who recovered fully, and your family and friends urge you to find some sort of job…well, you feel like you're betraying everyone when you don't get better.

My friend Daniel and his wife and daughter and I went out for dinner; this was a week or so before the holiday. My friends were flying abroad to visit friends of theirs, and so we would not be celebrating Thanksgiving together.

No sooner had we set foot in the restaurant than Heather started shrieking, "Sell your goddaughter to the gypsies! Beat the shit out of Daniel! Talk him into divorcing his wife! Why are you friends with these people? Be MY friend! They don't understand you! I know you! FUCK THEM!"

I heard Daniel's comments in snippets, but mostly I heard Heather and her little helpers:

"They're going to sell you out to terrorists."

"Call the cops and tell them Daniel is a criminal."

"I WANT THREE CHILDREN!" This of course was Heather.

"Sell your goddaughter to the Arabs."

"Daniel just slipped poison into your drink."

"Daniel's wife is reporting everything you say to the cops."

I was stunned. I had experienced a period of several weeks when the voices had been relatively quiet and most of my symptoms were paranoid delusions, but now the voices pounded back with a fury that stunned me. I could barely speak, and then only in short sentences, and I was horrified that some of this junk going on in my head would get out of my mouth and ruin my relationship with my friends.

On the ride home Daniel said, "Like I said last time we got together, you really should look for a part-time job. Having to deal with other people and do tasks that don't have anything to do with your illness will take your mind off your symptoms. It sounds weird, but a job will give you a break."

"I've been thinking of going back to volunteer at the library," I said hesitantly. "I don't know if I could do it or not, with these intense voices I'm experiencing. And Heather is hanging in there for the long run, I think."

"Daniel is right, you need to spend time around other people," his wife said. "A job would be good for you. Keep you healthy. *Socially* healthy."

The logic of their arguments was sound, but I knew they weren't getting what it was like to be in my head all day. When you read a mental illness memoir like this one, when Heather or the symptoms get too intense, or go on too long, you close the book and set it down and come back to it another day. I did not have this option. When Heather wanted to scream, she screamed, and sometimes that went on for four hours. There was no movie to turn off, no book to close, no remote control to change the channel. I got symptoms, all day every day, and they frequently drowned out everything that was going on around me. Work a job? HOW?

Reality, of course, was not on my side. A pleasant dinner with friends became a nightmare due to voices, and the beating wasn't over yet. A few days after the dinner, my computer began making a very loud noise, and then it overheated and shut down. I took it into the shop, where the tech said the cooling fan had broken, and it would take a few days to replace it. Having no choice, I gave him my laptop and took my receipt. I could not hunt for articles on mental illness, and I was reduced to going to the public library every few days to keep up with email on a library computer.

Also during this period, my feet kept hurting. I went and saw my primary care doctor, and he diagnosed me with plantar fasciitis. He prescribed a pair of inserts for my shoes, and I picked these up and tried them on. They felt a little weird, but I kept using them. Now I had two medical conditions ongoing.

Thanksgiving came along, and I went to the Salvation Army Thanksgiving dinner at Golden Hall. There were hundreds of people waiting to get in, maybe even a thousand people, in one line for people with kids or physical disabilities and one line for the rest of us. I stood there, restless and bored, when an elderly white man with a basset hound ambled up next to me and introduced his dog.

"His name is Bentley," he said, and the dog stared at him inquisitively. "What's your name?" the old guy asked.

The dog howled, and the people around him laughed.

The old guy kept up a string of patter: "He's a smart dog; he comes running as soon as he hears a can opener. He can always tell where the goodies are. I should get him a job as a politician, chasing the money."

"It's *your* money they're going after," hissed Heather, in my ear.

Who's going after my money? I thought at her.

The old guy said, "He's an old dog, and I'm an old man, and we have the same aches and pains. I take him for a walk every day, and he knows that after the walk comes the chow. He's not stupid; he knows where it's at. What comes after the walk, Bentley?"

The basset hound howled, and everyone laughed.

"T-4 Program," said Heather. "It's coming to America. First the Nazis declare everyone on disability to be a degenerate and a fraud and a parasite. Then they stop all disability payments. When you end up out on the streets, they send the SS around to herd you onto cattle cars and take you out into the desert. Guess what happens there?"

This freaked me out, because it seemed possible. It was no coincidence that lawmakers had been making comments against disabled people for the past few years, including president-elect Trump mocking a disabled reporter. They were lining it all up, finding supporters, looking for the people who were willing to carry out the next mass extermination. All that was now required was for the president-elect to pull the pieces together. Hitler's extermination orders against Germany's disabled people were signed in secret and carried out on the sly. More than a quarter million mentally and physically disabled Germans were murdered in a few years.

And of course, there were the cops, to see that the disabled were rounded up and sent off.

"You all right?" asked the old guy with the dog, looking at me. "You look kind of freaked out."

At that moment I was sure, dead certain, that I was going to end up as a naked corpse in a mass grave, somewhere out in the desert. Was this paranoia? Or politics? Or paranoia and politics feeding on each other?

"I'm really hungry," I mumbled.

"Bentley's hungry, too," he said, and the hound looked up at him. "How hungry are you, boy?"

The basset hound howled, and everyone laughed.

The line started moving, and I was surprised at how fast it went. In twenty minutes we were inside. A Salvation Army volunteer seated me at one of the long tables, and the old guy and Bentley sat next to me. There were about thirty people per table, seated close to each other, and the murmur of all the conversations of a thousand people messed with my head. Heather kicked up, not quite distinct, and I tried to focus on the people around me and ignore her.

The old guy seated next to me talked about the dinner, and his hound, and what it was like to be old. He was about ten years older than me.

"You're not going to be able to hike, in ten years," Heather said, in my mind.

I see old people out hiking, I thought.

"Not difficult hikes," she asserted. "You'll have to stick to paved paths, or pansy hikes like Los Penasquitos Canyon."

I might be hiking when I'm ninety, I thought.

"This guy with the dog is a spy for the cops," she said.

This struck me as absurd, because I knew the cops were spies for Heather. *Is he an undercover cop?* I thought at her.

"Could be," she replied in a neutral tone.

"Seems like some years the Salvation Army people put on a great feast, and some years they skimp on the servings," said the old guy.

"This old guy is an asshole," Heather said. "All he does is talk about himself."

All most people do is talk about themselves, I responded.

"Not me," she claimed. "Mostly I talk about YOU."

Some volunteers came by with Styrofoam plates loaded with food, and the feast began. The old man slipped some turkey meat to Bentley, under the table, and the hound ate it eagerly.

"Is he a service dog?" I asked the old guy.

"Hard to tell which of us is more decrepit," he chuckled. "Maybe I should get a vest that says I'm his service human."

I laughed, and he gave the hound some more meat.

"Trump is going to start with disabled people, and he's going to move on to old people," Heather said in a vindictive tone. "All going to the extermination camps. Say hello to the Final Solution, cripple."

I can fight, I said.

"The cops are on Trump's side," she said smoothly. "The soldiers are on his side. You don't even have a gun. What are you going to fight with, harsh language?"

"Basset hounds are incredibly loyal," the old guy said. "I've had him for years, and he guards the house day and night. I know what people say about German Shepherds being the best guard dogs, but don't underestimate basset hounds."

Donald Trump is a mainstream Republican of the business sort, I said to Heather. *I have uncles who are the same way. They're not Nazis.*

"Better wake up, dumb fuck, before Trump's soldiers drag you off." She said it in a cold tone.

Can't you just enjoy the meal? I thought in frustration.

I employed CBSST techniques and pictured former Turkey Day dinners I had had, and for maybe six or eight minutes I had peace. The old guy talked with other people for most of this time, and then he came back to me. At the same time Heather started yammering at me again. I tolerated these assaults for maybe five minutes, then I finished my meal. The old guy and his hound were funny, but Heather was going to trash any conversation I tried to have.

"Good talking with you," I said to the old guy, and he nodded. I waved at Bently, under the table, and then I went home.

A day or two later the guy at the computer shop called to let me know my laptop was repaired. I retrieved it and was extremely pleased when it started up without warnings flashing and without the cooling fan sounding like an airplane engine roaring. Right away I sat down at my desk and sent emails to friends.

"The cops are monitoring your computer," Heather hissed. "They're in your email and on your web browser." Her voice seemed next to my right ear.

"What are they looking for?" I asked her in frustration. She had ruined my dinner with Daniel and his family, and she had trashed my Salvation Army dinner. I couldn't tell where the cops really were, or what they wanted, but I didn't want to be savaged by deep paranoia.

"They are looking at *you*," she replied. "Evidence of wrong doing in the past, intent to perform crimes in the future. Hell, they don't even need to *find* evidence: the San Diego Police Department has a whole team who *manufacture* evidence on demand. Every police department in the country does evidence manufacturing."

The icy fingers of paranoia dug deep into my guts. Everyone

knew the cops falsify evidence. They give false testimony in court, and they pay off 'informers' who tell whatever story the cops tell them to provide. Cops plant drugs on suspects and lead witnesses to the 'right' story to tell.

"They won't have to make up stories," I said fearfully. "All they have to say is, 'he's mentally ill,' and that justifies *anything*."

There I sat on my battered old chair, at my desk, trying not to crap myself, because I *knew* the score. All those police cars on patrol past the café, the police foot patrols outside the grocery store, the security guards at the library giving me the eye…it was like a literary story where the author was foreshadowing the violence that was on the way.

The paranoia and hallucinations at the Salvation Army dinner disturbed me, and I decided I would take the initiative and try to get control of my illness. I typed up a list of all the symptoms I had experienced over the last year or so. The first dozen were easy, but as I kept describing symptoms, more and more popped up in my memory. Pretty soon I had twenty listed, and I was sure there were more. The list included Heather, in her own category, and hallucinations of homeless people, and paranoid delusions like thinking the cops were after me, and delusions of grandeur like thinking I was secretly worth a billion dollars. Some symptoms had stayed with me a few weeks or a few months, and some, like Heather, had been with me since the beginning.

Over the next few days I finished adding to the list, until there were 26 items in all. And some of those items were classes of symptoms with half a dozen sub-symptoms under them.

I sat at my desk and stared dumbly at the print-out as the full extent of my illness came home to me. Dozens of symptoms in an illness that had dragged on for ten years, with reprieves here and there that always gave way to extraordinarily bad times that went on for months. It seemed like the only way I was going to beat schizoaffective disorder was to step in front of a trolley.

I sent out an email to several friends, discussing how Daniel and his wife had urged me to find a part-time job. It didn't take long for them to respond.

One of my lady friends, Jackie, who is herself bipolar but has a job, said: "Go back to work? And what do you do when Heather starts yelling, and you can't perform your assigned tasks? Or are you supposed to sit there whispering, 'shut up' at the voices over and over? How could your employer keep you on the job?"

Another lady friend had a similar opinion: "See it from the employer's point of view. There's a ten year gap in your employment history. Why? Because you've been severely mentally ill. But you feel a little better now, so you'd like to go back to work. What's in it for you is a job, colleagues to talk with, the esteem of society for toughing it out, and some income.

"But what is the employer getting? Someone who can only work half time, who is subject to frequent attacks of mental illness, whose skills are ten years out of date and will need training, and who will say weird things on a frequent basis that will upset or alarm fellow workers. Why on earth should that employer hire you?"

"Some of my friends seem to think I'm well enough for a part-time job," I said to her. I felt like a fool, because I already knew she was right, but Daniel and his wife got my sense of hope up, and now that false hope was slamming hard into the reality of my situation.

"Do these people—the ones trying to get you to go back to work—do they run their own business?" my friend asked. "It's easy for them to talk, easy to recommend you go screw up someone else's business, but can *they* afford to accommodate your illness and pay you a living wage? Or are they psychiatrists who understand your illness inside and out? I think your friend's wife tipped her cards when she said you're just a parasite taking their money."

That got me thinking about what it was like at the café most mornings, with the conversations of the patrons setting off voices in my mind. How would I hold down a job in an office with dozens of colleagues all over the place? There would be land line phones ringing, cell phones chiming, computers beeping, colleagues talking at me all day, and a constant chatter of conversations that set off Heather and the minor voices.

I tried to put it all together, and here is what I got: some of my friends thought I should toss my hobbies and sit in a booth in a parking garage half the day and punch tickets. This would bring me something like eight dollars an hour, four hours a day. One hundred and fifty dollars a week, six hundred dollars a month. That wasn't enough to live on, and I'd still be mentally ill and on SSDI. So what would be gained by doing this? Placating my friends, to whom ten years of severe mental illness somehow looked like one long party?

Other friends were pretty sure that *any* job I took would be a disaster, and it was foolish to go back to work until I was really well. Jackie and I had another discussion, and she said, "What if you get into a work environment with a lot of stress? What is going to happen with your illness? Heather is going to go berserk. And you know, you could say something *really* weird, or Heather can get control of your mouth for two minutes, and *wham*, you lose your job and security escorts you out of the building...*or even worse*, you end up at the psych ward for six months, with guess who paying the bill?" In short, there were many ways to fail, and almost no way to succeed, in this matter of holding down a part-time job.

Sleep disturbances continued. I would sleep for a few hours and then wake up, over and over. Sometimes, just to break the monotony, I ate a snack or drank some fruit juice, and frequently I walked in circles around my room until I wore myself out and went back to sleep. I knew this was some manifestation of mania, and there was nothing to do but suffer these bouts of insomnia.

Near the end of the month I had a burst of curiosity in this matter of the president-elect promising to crack down on disability fraud. I went online and looked up "disability fraud" in a search engine, and the results were incredible. There was the "blind" man who was caught driving a car, and the doctor who faked a number of medical claims for people who wanted to receive SSDI; the doctor received a share of the disability benefits that these people were awarded. There were cases when people claimed to be disabled but actually worked a job, or two jobs, while receiving benefits. I could not see *anyone* disagreeing with cracking down on these blatant examples of fraud.

I continued to cruise the message boards on mental health sites on the web. There were a large number of people talking about their mental illnesses: bipolar and schizophrenia were common, and schizoaffective disorder came up from time to time. On one of these sites was a forum with news articles of interest to mentally ill people, and I looked at some of these. There was an article about mental illness in prison, and it was a horror story. For 2012 there were about 35,000 mentally ill people in state psychiatric hospitals in the U.S.. For the same year, there were 350,000 mentally ill people in prison in the United States.

In short, prisons have become a major provider of psychiatric care, and they often fall short in this role. Mentally ill prisoners often do not get the care they need, and they attack other prisoners, end up in solitary, do themselves harm, and sometimes kill themselves. Or they attack guards and are killed that way.

I read through this article several times, and I thought about the article I read months before, about mentally ill people being 16 more times more likely than someone without mental illness, to end up dead in an encounter with the police. That lead me to remember the article about 250 mentally ill Americans being killed every year, again by police.

The news was not good, but there was a tiny point of light, if you cared to look for it: a congressman named Tim Murphy, from Pennsylvania, introduced H.R. 2646: Helping Families in Mental Health Crisis Act, which proposed to reorganize mental health care in America. The legislation provided more money for community mental health centers, funding for psychiatric hospitals, and so forth. The deficiencies in the current system had been noted, and people at the highest levels of power were allocating money where it was needed.

At this point I had an epiphany: I was one of "these people," the journalists talked about. One of "these people" the cops routinely killed or threw in prison. One of "these people" that some lawmakers called a "drain on the economy." In short, the mentally ill had become a distinct class of people. There were ten million severely mentally ill people in the United States, and there were tens of millions more with a mild case of mental illness that would come to an end with proper medicine and therapy. We had detractors, and we had defenders, and it seemed that we had arrived on society's radar. In short, I was not just some guy who was half out of his mind; I was part of a large group of people whose advocates were developing some real social, political, and economic muscle.

To seal this recognition, I created an account with one of the mental illness web sites and began to talk to other people in the same situation as me. I posted links to all sorts of articles, about politics and mental illness, about medicines, about talk therapy and cognitive therapy, and about the relationship of the mentally ill and the cops. It seemed to me that there was a concerted effort to get rid of the mentally ill. Lawmakers called out the mentally ill as "parasites," and then the cops shot those people or threw them in jail, where they deteriorated further.

Of course Heather couldn't resist: "It's probably your fault that you're mental in the first place. What's wrong with working in a ticket booth for a few years? It's not important *what* you do, it's important that you make your friends happy. You don't have the backbone to stand up for yourself. Hell, I hope the cops shoot you. Or, you know…you could consider taking on the cops."

At this point I felt a strong burst of hostility toward the cops, *any* cops, and I wondered where the hell this came from. Then the term I was looking for popped into my head: asymmetric warfare. The kind of warfare where the two sides have radically different tactics, or one side is much larger than the other, or one side is better armed than the other, and so on.

I was in the middle of an asymmetric war between the cops and the mentally ill, and my side was losing. Someone had to take it upon themselves to even things up.

"How are you going to do that, dumbass?" Heather asked.

I didn't know, and she didn't give me any ideas.

December: nothing but a murderer

The holiday season hadn't been very good so far, and December started out with me trying to figure out where I fit in to the picture of mental illness in America. A few days into the month I had another paranoid hallucination of attacking a pair of cops on foot patrol, and in this fantasy I ended up dead.

"You don't even *have* knife-fighting skills," Heather jabbed, as I walked my daily exercise route. "You have skills at being stupid. You have skills at being pathetic. You listen to any advice your friends give you, because you have identified yourself as a cripple, and that means you believe you're a victim. Now pull your head out of your ass and listen: cops carry *guns*. Two cops, two guns. You come up from behind them and pull one of their guns and kill them both. Happens all the time."

The anticipation of easy victory coursed through my veins, and I looked forward to bringing some asymmetric warfare back to the source: the cops.

"Of course," she mused, "It could be you would fumble the gun, and the cops would put you in a choke hold and strangle the life out of you. In fact, given how fucked up you really are, I bet that's what would happen."

"My people need a champion," I said.

She had nothing to say to that, and I finished my walk in peace.

The temperature cooled down a few more degrees, and the air became crisp. I spent time looking up comments made by Donald Trump about his plans for disability, trying to pin him down. Some commentators said Trump was a supporter of SSDI, while his advisors were for gutting it. The president-elect himself said he was all for disability benefits for those who were truly disabled, but that the system was rife with fraud and needed weeding out.

I figured that journalists and opinion writers and political sharp-shooters were trying to squeeze the max dose of worry and fear out of the comments Trump had made; all the better to keep citizens running back to the media to find out the latest bad news. And commentators on social media said anything they pleased, an inane verbal diarrhea that their followers lapped up and asked for more.

It occurred to me to find out the *real* definition of disability, straight from the source: the Social Security Administration. The definition was easy to find, and here it is:

"Disability" under Social Security is based on your inability to work. We consider you disabled under Social Security rules if:

- You cannot do work that you did before;
- We decide that you cannot adjust to other work because of your medical condition(s); **and**
- Your disability has lasted or is expected to last for at least one year or to result in death.

I had already had conversations with my friends about my illness and the limitations it placed on my life. We had discussed what kind of work I might be able to do, and whether it was worth it to even try a part-time job. Could I convince an employer to take a chance on me to start with? Hell, I had paranoid delusions when I just sat still in my room, with no pressure on me, and Heather showed up when she pleased.

I was satisfied that I fit the criteria for disability, and I really didn't think that after ten years of schizoaffective disorder, I was going to get well all of a sudden. Somehow this realization gave me energy, and over the next few days I went to online mental illness forums and posted messages about stigma against mentally ill people, psychiatric drugs and their side effects and efficacy, cognitive behavioral social skills training, and what my symptoms were like. I read up on symptoms other people had experienced and was amazed at the incredible variety of delusions, hallucinations, paranoia, and so forth that mentally ill people experienced. Everyone had their stories: ending up in the psych ward after a full psychotic episode, thrown out of their parents' house after saying bizarre things to other family members, homeless, ruinous spending sprees, and other experiences of this sort.

"They're making all this up," said Heather, as I breathlessly read the posts on the forums.

"Why would anyone go online and leave a fake message claiming they're fucked up in the head and can't hold down a job?"

"Some people just like sympathy," she said.

"There are easier ways to get sympathy," I asserted. "I want to find out where I fit into the spectrum, and to warn those who have just come down with SZA about what they can expect."

"No one is going to match your exact symptoms," she said. "Why does everything have to be about you?"

Sometime around the second week of the month I started reading mental illness memoirs written by people who were schizoaffective like me. Due to my illness I was a slow reader, but most of these sorts of memoirs were short, and I made good progress. The author of one memoir had had run-ins with the law, DUI and that sort of thing. It had been years since the cops had seized my pistol and my car, and I hadn't really had any negative encounters with law enforcement in a long time.

"Sixteen times more likely to die," Heather whispered. "Two hundred and fifty mentally ill people a year."

Something had to be done.

My friend Steve and I went hiking at Tecolote Canyon Natural Park, an 8 mile trek on easy terrain. I wanted to tell him about the cops, and the asymmetric war, but I was afraid I would sound like a lunatic. We walked to a small park at the far end of the route and ate sandwiches, then we spent a few minutes bird-watching. We talked about short stories and novels we were reading. Eventually we returned to the nature center at the entrance of the park, and I walked to the trolley station and went home.

All that day, Heather was quiet. The minor voices kept their ugly comments to themselves. I knew the cops were hunting for me, eager to get some pistol practice. A paranoid vision popped into my mind, of a bored-looking cop talking with some reporters:

"Thing is, we *had* to shoot him," said the cop. This guy didn't look like a police chief, or spokesperson…just a regular cop who had somehow drawn the short straw in having to deal with the media. "He didn't respond to our commands, and he began yelling at us about asymmetric warfare. Turns out he was an infantry soldier, a long time ago."

A young female Asian reporter asked, "Was he armed?"

"He had something in his hands, but we couldn't see it clearly. It turned out to be a plastic bottle of water, but we didn't know that at the time. We told him to drop the weapon, and instead he rushed us. The rest was self-defense."

There was my entire war against the cops, summed up in twenty seconds. Fighting stupid, fighting symptoms, fighting for my people.

My mother called, and she sounded calm and precise as she said, "Your dad's cancer came back, about a week ago. The brain tumor, that is. The doctor said that the only measures left to fight it run a risk of causing permanent damage. Your dad could end up paralyzed, or lose the ability to speak, or fall into a vegetative state and not come out again. He could die outright.

"Your dad thought it over, and he decided not to keep fighting. He's been miserable for so long, and in such pain, that he just can't keep going. The doctor gave him two to four weeks. You really should come see him."

"Maybe it would be good if I talked to him now," I said.

"He's sleeping. That's what he does most of the time."

"I'll look into flying back there," I said, and we hung up.

Heather said, "You know those studies botanists conducted, where people watered their houseplants every day but otherwise ignored them? And then there was a group of people who watered their plants every day, and talked to their plants, too? And what happened? When the owners talked to their plants, the plants thrived. The other group of plants just did so-so.

"Do you get it? Your dad isn't dying of cancer. He's dying of your stupidity and negative thoughts. You don't talk to him enough, and when you do it's always about your little problems: your mental illness, your plantar fasciitis, your poverty. Asshole. You're a murderer. His cancer is a symptom of your neglect."

On the face of it, it seemed clear that this wasn't true. You didn't get cancer from "negative thoughts" or failure to chat often enough. Heather was on the attack again, trying to lay a guilt trip on me.

I wasn't sure what to do. My dad had been through tough fights with his cancer before, and he had always come out on top. Maybe he'd pull out of it this time, too. Maybe he'd beat the cancer for good and live another twenty years? In which case all this worry and stress was for nothing. Should I bet on my dad's stamina, or on the doctor's prognosis?

I went back and forth for a couple days: stay home, or go visit my parents? I called Daniel and told him the situation, and he said, "To me, there is only one choice here, and that's go visit your dad. It doesn't matter how much the plane tickets cost. Family is more important than money. *Maybe* he'll beat the cancer, but if he doesn't, you don't want to miss your last chance to talk with him."

These comments made me wonder if my dad really was going to die. What could I do to help him, or my mother? My father wasn't that old, in his seventies, and I guessed the pain had worn him down. He was ready to move on.

If I didn't go, and he died, I would feel guilty for the rest of my life. Daniel was right: in this no-win situation, family was more important than money.

I went to a travel site on the web and bought plane tickets for a few days in the future. I called my mother with the details, and she said, "Your father has gotten worse. He's slipping away. He sleeps most of the time, and even if you get here soon, he may be gone. I'll arrange for someone to pick you up at the airport."

Around the twentieth of December I went to the café in the afternoon and stood in line. Heather showed up in my mind, standing off to the left of me in summer clothes—loose blouse and cut-off shorts—that showed a lot of skin. She looked either miserable or drunk.

A young black man worked the register, and as soon as Heather saw this, she turned her head to face me. She looked gleeful.

"Hold my drink," she said, and though she wasn't holding a drink, I knew what she meant: she was about to do something stupid.

"NIGGER!" she bellowed. "GODDAMNED JIGABOO!!"

Horror was all I could feel. I swear, my heart gave a great lurch and stopped beating.

Uh… I thought at her.

"BRING BACK THE SLAVE DAYS!" she hollered, and I *knew* everyone could hear everything she said. But they would say *I* said it.

A few moments went by, and my heart started beating again. I realized the line had kept moving, and I walked up to the front and ordered a cup of coffee. The young man on the register gave no sign of having heard Heather, but that was just a front. Everyone was in on the "prank."

Shut the fuck up! I thought at her.

She saw a heavy-set woman sitting at a table, and she yelled, "FAT FUCK!"

I gingerly crossed the room and sat down and read for a while. Heather continued to shout slurs, as people walked by my table: race, gender, body type, and social class were all targets. I considered getting up and leaving the café, but what would that do except show Heather how she could get me to give up my favorite activities and run away?

"You'll *run*," she said. "Or I'll keep at you until you open your mouth and shout this crap at every person you see."

I read a few pages and felt that was all I could accomplish for that day, so I walked home.   All the way back, Heather and the minor voices took turns running people down and barking out more slurs. I felt awful that my dad was on his way out, and I trusted my mother's relatives to help her through his final days.

The next morning my mother called: "I can only talk for a few minutes; I have a lot of calls to make today. Your dad died yesterday. We had most of the arrangements worked out in advance, but there's still so much to do." She gave me the details: funeral, burial, who all was expected to come to pay their respects, who was coming to pick me up from the airport.

"So my last visit with dad is posthumous," I said. "I wish he could have held on for a few more days."

"Only God can decide that," she said. "See you when you get here."

On the cusp of Christmas I flew across the country and met up with my mother and some of her relatives, who drove us to my parents' place.

For the next few days relatives came to visit and tell stories about my dad. I recalled a few dumb but funny things dad and I had done together, such as the time I wanted to take a picture from the top of a cliff, at the Grand Canyon. This was when I was about ten years old.

"I don't think I can get a good shot from here," I said.

"Try this," my dad said, and he grabbed me by the back of the belt. "Lean out there, son."

I leaned way out over the cliff and took a shot straight down.

"Whoops, my grip is slipping. Lean back," he said.

I leaned back, and that ended that death-defying experience.

When my aunts and uncles told their own stories about my dad, I felt more connected to him. He wasn't dead, just moved on. One of my relatives reminded me that my grandmother—dad's mom—had died a few years ago, and so my dad wouldn't be lonely in heaven.

This did wonders for my state of mind, and I wished dad well in his new home. From time to time I felt sure that he wasn't really dead but was living in a five star hotel somewhere, surrounded by young Asian beauties from the movie industry.

Christmas was a strange holiday without my dad, and I felt a peculiar emptiness. My brother arrived, and in an attempt to fight this sense of loss, I said to him, "What was one thing you got from dad?"

"You mean, stuff?" he asked. He lives in Wisconsin and owns a house in a small town. From time to time he gets into fitness and does kick-boxing, or karate, and activities like that.

"For example, dad got me interested in the American Indians," I said. "And there were all those parks we visited, when we were growing up. Grand Canyon, Grand Tetons; like that. I still enjoy hiking. I'm still into the Indians. Hell, I got a masters degree in anthropology. That was dad's influence."

He smiled and patted his stomach. "Beer belly. Dad's was bigger, but I've still got twenty years to work on mine."

We laughed, and I slapped my own pot belly in response.

Heather said, "You're nothing but a murderer. You're making fun of the man who sired you, who raised you and got you on your way in life. You're a real asshole, you know that?"

It's Christmas, Heather. Why don't you take a break?

"I'm going to keep it up, until you take responsibility for your actions. Murderer!"

A couple days after Christmas we went to the funeral. About thirty people came and paid their respects. Before the service began, Heather belted out a mocking version of "Another One Bites the Dust," which is a song by the group Queen. Then she repeated it, over and over, through the service and the viewing of my father's corpse. What could I do? If I told her to shut up, or knock it off, she'd just intensify her attacks, and the situation would become worse. I decided to concentrate on showing my respects to my dad, and I put up with Heather the whole way.

We drove with my dad to the cemetery, and a two-man military honor guard presented the flag to my mother. The other guard played taps, and the sad notes of that tune seemed directed at me. All of a sudden it sank in on me that my dad was really dead and that I would never see him again in this world. I thought of my walk to Cancer Survivor's Park, just a few months ago, when I wondered if my dad would win or lose this current bout of cancer. The coffin in front of me was a shocking answer to that query.

My heart broke, and I cried for my dad, and for the rest of us as well, who would one day meet our maker.

"Sure," Heather hissed in my ear. "Blame it on the *cancer*. You know whose fault it is. Just keep broadcasting hate and stupidity. You'll kill the whole planet!"

The burial detail lowered my dad's coffin into the ground and filled in the grave. The question I had asked a month or two ago, about which one of us—my father or me—would die first due to our medical condition had been answered.

The next day some of my relatives took me the airport, and a few hours later I was home again.

The last few days of December were melancholy. My dad had come to his end, the year had come to its end, and Heather stabbed my heart with thorns of misery. She heaped on the racial and sexual slurs as soon as I left my room in the morning and she kept these going during my morning walks. I began to hate her, in part for the ugly comments and in part because I was sure she was going to blame her slurs on me.

Of course, I knew that all this came back around to the cops, one way or the other. One morning I went to the café, and Heather said, "I've made up a song for you; it's called 'The Song of Authority.' It's for all those district attorneys and judges and cops out there, gaming the system and getting away with murder. In fact, something like that could happen to *you*. Here's the song:

"Our boys in blue, right or wrong;

Our boys in *blue*, right or wrong;
Our *boys* in *blue*, **right** or **wrong**;
Our boys in blue! **RIGHT!** Or **WRONG!**

"I'm not much of a poet, but it says what we all know. You should type it up and post it on social media."

"I'd rather—" I started, but she cut in with,

"Who killed your dad? If it wasn't you, who was it? I think we both know the answer to that one."

And I *did* know who: it was the cops. Not directly, no, but it was like secondhand cigarette smoke: not direct, but lethal nonetheless. The cops carried out their war on the mentally ill, and the bodies filled the graves. My dad was not a fool: he had seen that my turn would come. The cops must be watching me every day, waiting for any little deviation from my usual routine, looking for a chance to kill me. My dad had known that my days were numbered, and the stress of this knowledge wore him down and fed the cancer and killed him.

I went to the café and read a chapter from a book, then I went for a walk. My emotions were churned up, and maybe that was what caused Heather to say: "You see, your dad was pretty smart, and he passed that on to you. You've known the cops are looking to kill you, all along. Subconsciously. Question is, what can you do?"

"I'll cut their throats," I growled.

"Talked about this one already. And shooting them with their own guns."

As I recalled, both these ideas ended up with me dead. "What do *you* have to contribute?" I asked.

She chortled, "Ask yourself this: what's the price of pork?"

I went ten or eleven blocks up the street, then crossed over to the next street and walked back. When I arrived home, I sat down in front of my computer and looked up media stories on mental illness and homelessness. I found an article that laid down this statistic: there are six hundred thousand homeless people in the United States. One in five of these people are severely mentally ill. Was it any wonder some of them got in trouble with the cops?

"I decided to have a party, and you're the guest of honor," Heather laughed.

I heard boots tromping on the floor downstairs, and the crackle of radios as police charged up the stairs. It had been a while since I had experienced this sort of hallucination, and I have to admit that every muscle in my body tightened up.

"I don't have a gun," I pleaded with Heather.

"Just keep your shit together," she said. I couldn't see her; she was just a voice that day.

"Who the fuck you be?" someone from downstairs asked, very loudly. I didn't hear a response from the police.

Boots ran up the stairs, and then Heather left, but her voice was loud from outside my door: "Gentlemen! A friend of mine has a story for you," she said.

"What kind of a story?" belted one of the cops.

"It goes like this: say it, Randal."

The cops and Heather were in the hall, and I sat at my computer desk and wished for an assault rifle. Instead, all I had were words, so I called out in a loud tone of voice: "When I was a boy, the police had two functions. One, they promoted public safety, like 'always wear floatation devices when boating,' or 'remember to buckle up when in a vehicle.' Two, catch criminals and put them in prison.

"Forty years went by, and the police still have two functions, but those functions are now: to kill mentally ill people, and to seize citizens' assets.

"My question is, who changed? Did the citizens of the United States get deeper into blood sport, or was it the cops who thought it would be more fun to hunt disadvantaged people and grab everything of value they could get hold of?"

"We all changed," said a cop, outside my door. I couldn't see him, but if he and his colleagues came bursting through the door I'd get a big eyeful of him, because it sounded like he was in front of the pack. He continued talking: "You didn't go back far enough in time. It was losing the war in Vietnam that made everyone into an asshole.

It was supposed to be an easy war and an easy victory, and we lost it and began to doubt ourselves. To compensate, Americans have been more aggressive ever since."

"That actually makes sense," I said.

There came a loud slamming on my door, and I stood up and prepared to die. I was in a state beyond fear, so freaked out that my heart couldn't even respond by beating too fast. Heather didn't fool me. It might be cops at my door, but she had goaded them on. She had arranged this whole thing.

I opened the door and found an empty hallway. No cops, no one at all; this whole episode was some sort of hallucination/delusion. I stepped out into the artificial light and looked around.

"This has to stop," I said to Heather, but she had done her thing for the day and had gone to wherever she went when she wasn't plotting against me.

That was how I ended 2016: my father had died, Heather and the cops were after me, and I was still barking mad and getting a little more paranoid and angry each day.

January 2017: asymmetric warfare

The new year started off with me reading more mental illness memoirs. All of these works focused on schizoaffective disorder, and many of the symptoms their authors experienced were similar to my own. It did not surprise me that spending weeks and weeks digging deep into this illness triggered my own symptoms, and I kept experiencing flashbacks as I read the books. This was unpleasant, but I wanted to take this journey with other mentally ill people and see how they handled their own symptoms.

As a result, I gained a strong sense that these men and women, these mental illness sufferers, were my people. They had taken the journey into madness, and they had survived and reported back to the rest of us what they had found in the darkness. Some of them had been committed to psychiatric wards, voluntarily or against their will, and some of them had been arrested and thrown in jail because their illness made them do weird things. Thoughts of suicide floated in and out of their minds, and the voices they heard were as malevolent as Heather often was.

My people were fighting two wars at once; one of these wars was a daily battle against their symptoms, and the other was the war against the cops. Just last September an unarmed black man died at the hands of police in El Cajon, a small community near San Diego. The man had an object in his hands and pointed it at the police, who shot him dead. Later the cops found out that the man was mentally ill, and the object was a vaping device.

"This guy didn't fight hard enough," Heather chided. "He was sick enough to stand up to the cops, but he wasn't armed enough."

"You've pretty much convinced me that using a knife or a gun against the cops is suicide," I muttered.

"Don't sweat it, I'm working on an idea," she said.

"*You're* going to commit suicide?" I burst out with great excitement.

She stood next to me at my desk at home, annoyance on her face, but she then cocked her head and said, "You were a soldier once, ready to fight for your country. Remember that? Back when you were young? When you had a pair of balls and weren't a nutless loser?"

I gritted my teeth, and she barreled onward: "If you think about it, you'll know what to do," she said. Then she was gone, and I got on the computer and started sorting out various media articles that talked about the problems with mental illness in America. I posted messages about violence and mental illness to online forums and was amazed when only two or three other people replied to my posts. Why the hell didn't anyone want to discuss violence against the mentally ill? You don't convince the cops to change tactics by ignoring the problem.

As I dug around, I found an article that changed the way I saw problems with mental illness and violence. USA Today ran the piece, and it was entitled, "40,000 suicides annually, yet America simply shrugs." According to the article, people with mental illness account for 90% of all suicides in America; this is a hundred suicides a day, *every day of the year.*

This sad statistic stunned me, and the article put mentally ill violence in terrible perspective. There were mentally ill people like Jared Loughner and James Holmes and Adam Lanza, who lashed out at society and killed a few people, and then there was this terrible toll of suicides by the mentally ill. When you talk with your friends, your family, and interested strangers about mental illness, everyone will bring up the mentally ill murderers. You rarely hear the stories of the mentally ill people who commit suicide.

As I read the article, I thought about how the game is rigged, right here in the good old USA. Lawmakers shut down psychiatric hospitals all across the nation, citing high operating costs, and the mentally ill people were dumped on the streets and told to use community mental health centers on an outpatient basis. For the higher-functioning mentally ill people, this system more or less worked, but many severely mentally ill people couldn't cope. Most of the people in this condition ended up homeless or in prison, where they are at the mercy of the elements and hard-core criminals. Or, of course, they died at the hands of the police.

My understanding of the situation of the mentally ill in America changed. The asymmetric war that I had envisioned was more widespread than I had thought. Lawmakers and jailors worked with politicians to deny care, close down housing, and turn mental health issues into law enforcement issues. And if a politician suggested their state, or their city, or their county, allocate more funds for mentally ill services, they were quickly shouted down on the grounds that if the government made more money available for mental health care, all that would happen is that more mentally ill people across the country would get on the bus and come to where the care was. The problem would never be solved; it was simply a matter of moving sick people from A to B and letting someone else deal with it.

My friend Kevin and I got together for brunch at a restaurant near my place. I told him about this research I was doing. He is a lecturer at a local university, and he is bipolar. His condition is under control, with the meds easing his symptoms.

"I bet you, the deeper you dig, the angrier you're going to get," he said. "I visit my shrink on a regular basis, call him if there's any change in the illness, and take my pills, like a good little boy. It works for me."

"It's incredible what is going on," I said. "Thirty-six *thousand* mentally people commit suicide every year."

"Are you thinking about checking out, too? Why are you so intense about this?"

"As I read this stuff, I get this strong feeling that these are my people. America has declared war on my people."

"Send a letter to the editor of the paper. Let your voice be heard!"

What I felt like was killing some people, to make a point. But I didn't know which people would make the best examples. Who should I finger?

"I'm on this online forum," I said. "The people who post there are more mentally fogged than angry. Mostly they're trying to get through the day. They post about losing jobs or being unable to work, or they say a few words about how their parents kicked them out, and now they're living out of their car or out of a tent. Lots of people post about their meds or their therapists. I seem to be the only one talking about violence and mental illness."

"Be careful on those forums," Kevin said. "Don't use your real name. All these people are mentally ill, and some of them are really disturbed. Not just a little depressed, but believe they are talking to God and He's telling them to kill you."

"Yeah," I said. "I wanted to run this past you; it's a print-out of an experience I had in Las Vegas back in 2008. I had a gun and nearly killed people. Really intense. I am thinking of posting it."

He took the sheet of paper and read it, then he said, "Wow, that's gripping. Those voices, they get to you."

"It was sheer luck of the draw that no one was injured," I said. "The voices fought it out, and the murderous voices lost. But it was really close."

"Do you have any weapons now?" he asked me.

"No," I blurted, then out came a spew: "Guns...no money... can't get enough money for shooting cops, protect myself... These cops say I'm crazy, but I'm not killing anyone...Why is it they call me...crazy? Why am I crazy? When did *I* kill...an unarmed...black man? What...about you?"

He stared at me and said, "Is that Heather, messing with your head?"

"She doesn't like guns," I said. "But she wants... to marry. She wants kids. She wants—"

"Wait a second. Is she paying your rent? Is she cooking your dinner? Does she listen to your problems? Why should you listen to her? Tell her to either help you out in a tangible way, or go to hell."

He said this without rancor, and for just a few moments I realized how miserable I was, being dominated by voices in my head. Voices from people I usually could not see, who did nothing for me whatsoever, who antagonized and aggravated day after day. The big promises had resonance just for being repeated so often: Nobel Peace Prize, a billion dollars, Presidential Medal of Freedom with distinction, British Knighthood, and of course, an end to the torment that dominated much of my life.

I wanted some explanation for what I had gone through. Either I was severely mentally ill, and all the psychiatrists and all the meds had had only a small effect on symptoms that had lasted for years… Or I was up to my eyeballs in a conspiracy carried out by hundreds or even thousands of people at all levels of society for more than a decade.

"We're making you mentally ill so we can give you a great life afterward. It's the future: everything good is in the future."

Heather, fuck off, I thought at her.

"Lover boy, you'll get your reward when I say you can have it. I think you're not serious about helping your people. You're not complaining about the situation of mentally ill people in America, you're complaining about me putting a little pressure on you."

"I've been down all the way, too," Kevin said. "Bipolar, forgetting to take my meds, homeless with fifty bucks in my wallet, wandering around New Mexico like a lost soul."

"Be glad you didn't hear voices," I said.

"Had my own version of hell," he said. "You've been there; you know the drill. Homeless steal from each other, they beat each other up, they have all sorts of run-ins with law enforcement. Cops put me in jail for being drunk, but I was bipolar, not drunk. Forgot to take my meds…"

We talked a while longer about living in culverts or beneath bridges, and then his parking meter was about to run out, so he said,

"I just pray I never end up that way again. It's like a war, where every day you might die. I don't know if I have the courage to go through that again."

"No, I'd step in front of the trolley if I became homeless again," I said.

We shook hands, and he left. I paid my bill and slowly wandered back to my room.

"You always complain about me," Heather groused.

"You're a symptom," I said. "Mental illness, or conspiracy?"

"You're probably too stupid to tell the difference," she said. "I don't enjoy conversations with your mentally ill friends. They're duller than you are."

"My friends just hope I will get rid of you," I said.

"I'd like to see that," she said in a mocking tone.

A few days went by. I enjoyed the cold weather and laughed at the images that some of my friends in Denver posted to Facebook, with two feet of snow on their yards. I went to see my psychiatrist at the VA hospital, and we discussed my symptoms.

"Your hands are shaking more than last time," she noted, so she took me off Risperidone and put me on Latuda, an anti-psychotic I had never even heard of before. I hoped it would do some good.

"Are you having thoughts of hurting yourself or others?" she asked me.

Constantly, I thought, but I figured that admission was a good way to get sent to the funny farm, and I said, "No."

"All right." Then we discussed the common side effects for Latuda, and she ordered me a batch of pills from the pharmacy. I picked up the pills and went on my way.

Her question about harm to myself or others dug in deep. How should I answer her? I figured that if I was self-aware enough to hedge my answers, that meant I was well enough to avoid harming anyone. If I was so lost in my psychosis that I would walk around telling people that I was planning to kill someone, didn't that mean I *should* end up in the laughing academy?

But I did talk about the war on my people. On the mental illness forums I posted messages about the mental illness topics that interested me most, and a few people posted tepid responses. Every day I felt more anger at the bad situation of my people, and yet it seemed I was alone in my views. Other people on the forums seemed to accept that the situation would never change, or that there was nothing they could do to stop the deaths.

It is time to discuss an incident where I almost killed a bunch of people. This is what I showed Kevin over breakfast; this is the event that I kept thinking about as I contemplated how to carry out a war on the cops. I didn't include this incident in my first memoir, because it used to really upset me even to think about it. Now years have passed, and the emotions are no longer so raw. The whole thing happened in early 2008, when my illness raged and I had not yet found my way into treatment. Ready? Here it goes:

I was in Las Vegas, Nevada, where I was homeless and living out of my car. The schizoaffective voices had been on me for days, urging me to escalate. I knew what the voices wanted: I was in possession of a 9mm pistol, and they wanted me to kill someone. Heather was not present; it was minor voices in a storm of hate. One morning during commute hour I parked at a gas station and slipped my pistol into a coat pocket. I got out of the car and sat down at the side of a major thoroughfare. For the next hour the voices screamed: "They'll kill you if you don't kill them first!" "You've *got* to kill them!" "Save yourself!" And on and on and on. I kept one hand on the pistol at all times, running my fingers over the cold metal and counting and re-counting the loose ammo. Forty rounds, in all. A lot of dead or wounded citizens.

The cars rushed past. Every minute or two the traffic light turned red, and all the cars stopped. They were packed in like sardines. The voices howled: "Just walk between the rows of cars, and kill the drivers! Kill their kids! Kill their passengers!" "They're CIA, and they're looking for you! They'll *kill* you!" I pulled the gun halfway out of my pocket and tried to determine which driver to kill first. It was clear that I had to kill the drivers of the cars in front first. That way, the cars behind them couldn't escape. Then I could kill *those* people, too.

Then a "friendly" voice came into my head, urging me to compassion. It was a female voice that sounded vaguely like my mother, and it said, "These people haven't hurt you. It's the bad voices that are hurting you. You don't want to shoot anyone. Except maybe yourself, and I forbid it."

Rush hour passed, and the flow of traffic decreased. The bad voices and the friendly voice shot comments back and forth at each other and argued their positions. I was helpless to take sides. I could neither leave the gas station nor start shooting, but I knew that if I sat on that curb for much longer, the gas station attendant would notice I had been there a while and ask me to move along. He'd probably be the first one I shot.

"Go in peace," said the friendly voice, and the bad voices were silent. I slid the gun back into my pocket and got into my car and drove away. About a week later the cops saw my car parked in a suspicious place, and they searched the vehicle and took the pistol.

Time passed. I found my way into treatment, and my life got better. I received SSDI, and my name was entered into a government database, so I couldn't buy any more guns.

So, I get it. I understand what happens with mentally ill men who turn murderous. They have the opposite outcome of my experience: the good voices lose, the bad voices win, and there is a massacre. The line between killing all those people or just driving away was so thin that it made me sweat just to remember it.

"Wow," Heather said, somewhere in my mind. "The question isn't, 'what happened back then,' but 'what will you do now?'"

"I came close to violence back in 2008," I said to her. There was a push-push feeling in my guts that meant Heather was going to urge me to do something I didn't want to do, and I said, "Why do you come around, anyway? I don't want you. I don't want your messages, and I don't like the 'help' you give me."

"Then come to Los Angeles and fuck me. When you give me what *I* want, I'll give you what *you* want. And, are you sure you didn't shoot those commuters? Maybe you're suppressing the memory."

This annoyed me, and I said, "Don't you think *maybe* someone would have noticed a guy with a pistol killing forty people?"

"Yeah, well, violence from 2008 doesn't interest me much anyway," she said impatiently. "What *interests* me is that deep down, you are a fighter. You're kind of pitiful at it, but you did the right things at the right time: procure weapon and ammo, scout out the massacre site, determine how the targets would react, and work up your courage to the event. If *I* had been there, you would have carried through. Next time I will be there. You're just trying to manage symptoms, and I'm way out in front, thinking of the next big event. Maybe something closer to home, this time?"

Of course, symptoms continued. My coffee breaks at the café began to depress me, because the illness ripped me off: my peace of mind, my ability to concentrate, my willingness to talk with friends and relatives. I could chalk up the losses: all the books I would have read if I didn't have voices in my head, the stories I would have written if I could concentrate, and the friendships I could have maintained if only I wasn't complaining so often about my symptoms. I could have developed my computer skills into a good career, if my mind wasn't full of noise all the time. The possibilities seemed endless. My illness was a thief, and it stole away a good life and replaced that good life with misery.

As I tallied the opportunity costs of schizoaffective disorder, I thought, *This has gone on too long.* Was I delusional all the time, or were my friends and family taking advantage of me in some weird conspiracy? Over the years I had sent hundreds of emails begging my friends and family to stop tormenting me, and the situation didn't improve. If complaining to the people who were holding me down wasn't working, what would?

"Seems like you need to kill some fuckers, show them you're serious," Heather offered, somewhere around mid-month. She caught me as I took a walk through the Gaslamp district.

She went on, "I have an idea, but you're not ready for it yet."

You're pissing me off, I warned her.

"I'll spill when you're ready for the idea of the century."

"Nuclear weapons?" I asked.

"See? You think you're funny, but all you're showing me is that you're fucked up in the head. Nukes? Bold, but the government probably guards those bad boys, don't you think?"

I walked down the Martin Luther King Jr. Promenade, which is a brick path next to the trolley tracks. The chill air felt good, but my thoughts returned again and again to the question, *what would it take to steal a nuke and drop it on Washington, D.C.?*

"Forget the nukes. Think, 'cops,'" she goaded.

"What do you want, Heather?" I snapped. "Spell it out."

"Just think about it."

An hour later I had finished my walk and went home, and I sat at the computer and searched for information on mental illness. The most frightening factoid I came across was on the website for CNN, where a psychiatrist named Charles Raison cited the "law of thirds," which applies to psychotic disorders. About a third of all people with psychotic disorders will recover and lead normal lives. About a third more will stabilize but will never recover. And about a third will not stabilize or recover but will decline.

As I absorbed this information, my heart pounded, and I felt dizzy. I wasn't in the downward spiral, but I wasn't recovering, either. I was in that group of psychotics who have stabilized, but the illness was there all the time, and every day was a fight. Should I wonder when the descent into hell would begin, or would it be wiser to place my bet on finding a useful medicine that would help me make a full recovery?

I came across an online article in the web site for *Time*, entitled: "After Aurora, Questions About Mass Murder and Mental Illness." One statistic in the article jumped out at me right away, that schizophrenics are nearly twenty times as likely to murder someone than a healthy person is.

Heather was not with me in vision, but her voice said, "Now you're going in the right direction. You're totally bugshit schizo, and society will harass you until you break; then they will kill you. I say, get them first."

"Get who first?" I grumbled, but I knew who. Who killed hundreds of my people every year and locked up the ones they didn't kill outright?

The cops.

As January went on, I posted sad notes on social media, about my dad's death and some of the life lessons I learned from him. Friends posted their condolences, and my closest friends offered a shoulder to cry on. Some of them shared their own losses with me, and it turned out that no fewer than five of them had lost a parent in the past few years. It was that time of life, when my cohort was in their forties and fifties, and our parents were passing away.

After a week of this, Heather said, while I shopped for groceries, "Cancer didn't kill your dad. We've been over this. *You* killed him. Your hateful thoughts caused the cancer in the first place, so you murdered him. That's *your* fault."

I thought you'd say it was the cops who killed him.

"The cops are like janitors; they clean up all the messes no one else wants to take care of. The cops kill everyone, in the end."

I went out to the mental health forums where I was a member and posted links to the news articles I had found, but the response was lackluster. This made me angry. Didn't anyone else see the patterns here? The media said that most mentally ill people were not violent, but then they jumped right into the shock statistics about murderous psychotics. All of American society was playing an elaborate game of "kill the mentally ill."

It seemed smart to read these articles carefully, over and over again, and to return to the ones that best fed my anger. At the same time, the minor voices kept up their attacks. Whenever I went online and saw a picture of a person of color, or a woman, on the news sites I was exploring, the minor voices screamed out racial slurs and gender attacks. This also took place with live people. Every time I went into the café, the voices screeched and snarled their insults. When police cruisers went by, Heather belted out,

"Here, piggy pig pig! What's the price of pork today?"

I didn't understand why I was hearing this crap, but I lived in terror that these noises would get out of my mouth and get me sued. This symptom hadn't occurred in earlier years of my illness. The only thing that changed was that my dad had died, and I was feeling a lot of sorrow for this loss and a lot of anger because America was demeaning, attacking, jailing, and killing my people.

On the 20th of January I started mumbling to myself in the café. This was early morning, and my mind was wound up like a motor.

"Who's the genius here?" I murmured. "If it's me, why don't I have more money? Cops. Everyone knows mentally ill people end up dead, but they're okay with that as long it isn't their loved ones who die." As I spoke, more anger came out in my voice. There weren't many people in the café this early in the day, but one of them glanced my way as I spit out, "I bet someone is ripping me off, right now. Getting ready to sell me to the cops. Snitches. Informants. They seize your assets. *Mother fuckers!*"

I recognized that my symptoms were about to run out of control, so I left the café and went straight home.

"No one knows if I'm a genius or not. Timothy McVeigh was a genius. I SHOULD KICK SOMEONE'S ASS! No one audits the fucking cops! THEY ARE UNACCOUNTABLE!" I was almost yelling, and I forced my mouth shut and stumbled home. In that small, chilly room I sat down and waited until I calmed down. Heather hadn't shown up in a day or two, and I could not blame this lapse on her. I was going back to the days of barking madness, when I was homeless and living on the streets of Santa Fe, New Mexico. That had been a dark and evil time, and it seemed I was going to return to those horrors.

Around this point in the month, I checked out a book from the library, entitled *Literary Genius.* There were twenty-five essays discussing the careers and works of literary geniuses from the last few centuries, and why those writers are considered geniuses. The introductory essay said that literary genius was defined as a *style* that was so groundbreaking and fresh that it made readers see their lives and their place in the world in a new way.

It didn't take me long to realize that I, too, "had to be" a genius. Didn't the criteria fit me exactly?

This "realization" that I was extremely bright and gifted made me even angrier, because what the hell were people doing to me? Fake mental illness and endless fake "problems" that wasted my potential and ruined my life! And who was responsible?

Heather, and the cops.

Every day when I went to the café, Heather shouted slurs at people of color, and women. The more this bothered me, the more frequently and more intensely she belted out her comments. Sometimes I found myself whispering these insults, as she tried to get me to shout along with her.

As she yelled, I would see my father laying in his coffin. His hands were crossed on his chest, and he looked at peace. I could not recall a single time he had slurred anyone, and I didn't understand the connection between him and Heather.

So I decided to throw it out to the mentally ill community and wrote up a post discussing this situation. A few people posted replies, where they discussed their own voices that howled out slurs, but this did not seem to be a common symptom.

This really puzzled me. There are an estimated ten *million* severely mentally ill people in the United States, including about five million people with psychotic conditions like schizoaffective disorder and schizophrenia. All those people experiencing symptoms, and only two or three heard racial slurs in their hallucinations? Or was this subject such taboo that everyone was afraid to admit their voices were that ugly?

Every day I checked back to this message, but no one new took on the subject.

It wasn't Heather who took me the next step toward violence; it was my own sense of belonging to a persecuted group. I was not a healthy person anymore, and I wanted to figure out who I belonged with.

Like a dream, there they were: Adam Lanza, Jared Loughner, James Holmes. As I looked up their stories on the web, these losers in the game of life, it seemed clear to me that these men felt persecuted, and they struck back. Were their actions political, or just an expression of their mental illness?

"You're superior to these guys," Heather said, in my mind. "They were just broke-dick losers, but you are seeing reality. You're a genius, and you're looking straight into deeper patterns that other people can't see."

"Heather, I *know* I'm mentally ill. But sometimes…"

"It's not paranoia if they're really out to get you," she said.

"These people were lone gunmen. They were not organized, and they did not stand for anything. They were not even fighting a war on cops, or society, or anyone. They were just sick in the head."

"I'm glad you realize you're better than them. I think it's time you contributed to the war."

"I agree."

"Well, that was easy! You gave up the knife attacks, and you gave up the pistols, and I think we can safely set aside loose nukes. What does that leave?"

"I can steal a car or an SUV—"

"There's a name you didn't look up. You imply you stand for something, that you're the face of the politics of mental illness. There was another guy who stood up for his politics, and he was very successful at it. Think on it, and I'll bet you remember his name."

In seconds a light went on in my mind, and I typed, "Timothy McVeigh" into the search engine. All sorts of information came back, and I started reading. On April 19, 1995, McVeigh detonated a truck bomb outside the Alfred P. Murrah Federal Building in Oklahoma City, Oklahoma. The explosion and building collapse killed 168 people and injured hundreds more. McVeigh, and a couple accomplices, fled the scene, but one of the accomplices turned himself in and gave up the name of the other men, and law enforcement soon arrested the other accomplice. Authorities caught McVeigh as he tried to get away, and they pieced together his story, which was a combination of radical politics, anger at the government, military training, and a willingness to fight.

"This guy kicked ass," I said to Heather.

"You said that mentally ill people are *your* people," she pressed. "Tim researched, planned, and carried out his fight for *his* people. He was political. He walked his talk. And some people say he was mentally ill.

"Every week the cops blow away a few more mentally ill people. But law enforcement has accomplices, and that is *you.* You allow this to go on. The cops have resources, weapons, and will to fight. You *talk* some shit, but when are you going to *fight?*"

Then she shut up. There I was, angry and admiring a man who fought for his convictions, knowing what should be done but lacking the will to do it.

For a few days I read about literary geniuses and fed my own genius. Part of this was sending out emails to friends and family, declaring my own genius and pointing everyone to an illustrated novel that I had written many years ago and had posted online.

"There is a problem with claims to genius," I said to my lady friend Jackie, in an email exchange. "In physics and mathematics, geniuses demonstrate their caliber by doing math that is beyond what everyone else can do. They just show you the math, and that proves it. In the literary sense, genius is more a matter of opinion. Some people argue that Jane Austen is a genius, and others argue she is not. Is Hemingway a genius? Some experts say yes, some say no. You have to present your work and convince the authorities that you have the right stuff. There is no definitive measure, like math."

"I have no idea if your work is proof of genius," she said, "But I looked at the illustrations in your book, and they're beautiful. You should look into publishing it."

As January closed out, I did more research on Timothy McVeigh, and one article I found listed the materials that he used to make his bomb. This seemed incredible; everything I needed to know about how to make the weapon was right there in black and white.

"The Feds know about this list," said a minor voice in my head. "They track all the people who access this web page. If you come back several times, they charge you with planning a terror attack."

I knew this had to be true. What the hell was the National Security Agency doing, if not sucking up all that information on extremists and compiling terror watch lists?

These pieces of mental illness and politics and violence began to cascade in my mind. The cops killed two hundred and fifty mentally ill people every year. Mentally ill people sometimes became violent and killed dozens of citizens. 36,000 mentally ill people a year committed suicide, and little was done to staunch the flow.

Timothy McVeigh had revealed the way I could follow: my military training, the recipe for a truck bomb on the internet, a rental truck, and an asymmetric war with a massive body count.

This sickling was going to fight back.

February: the victor

I had read several mental illness memoirs about schizoaffective disorder, and I had re-read my own memoir, and I started on an outline for this memoir you are reading now. Almost right away I started experiencing symptoms, as I read through old emails from the period I wanted to cover.

"Kill some cops!" urged a minor voice.

"Blow them all up!"

"Make it a murder-suicide!"

During times when the symptoms were severe, I played music, and this sometimes calmed the voices. Other times, music aggravated the symptoms and became another form of attack on my embattled mind.

I complained to friends about my symptoms and my suspicion that I was triggering my own illness.

My friend Steve said, "If you're making your illness worse, maybe you shouldn't work on this memoir. You could write a novel or some poetry or something."

"I figured it out, and it will take me about 3 months to write a rough draft of the whole memoir," I said. "That is, writing six days a week. That isn't so long."

"Maybe try a compromise," he suggested. "Take more days off from writing, and see if that makes a difference."

"I guess I could take two days off each week, instead of one. That would mean another month to get a draft together."

"It will be worth it if you don't have to listen to these voices so much."

What he didn't say, what *all* my friends didn't say, was that they didn't really want to hear more complaints about symptoms that I was triggering myself. This brought me frustration, because what should come first: my memoir, or my friends?

This compromise didn't work very well. I honored my part of the bargain and took more time off, but when I *was* working on the outline, the symptoms were harsh.

"The cops aren't smarter than you," Heather snapped, as I took a walk past police headquarters. "The cops want to *destroy* you people, and you have no idea how to even *fight*."

The bouquets that had festooned the monument to fallen officers were all gone now, and as I went on my way I noticed structural supports that held up the headquarters building. I chewed over possible problems getting the rental truck into place, and I noticed how many cops were around the front of the building. I sketched out a plan in my mind, for how to blow up the building and kill two hundred cops.

"How are you going to escape, once you get the truck in place?" Heather asked. "Details! Details!"

"I can… I can use a…um…"

"Remote control from an aerial drone," she said happily.

I couldn't figure out why she was so excited about this, and that distracted me. A police cruiser went by, and I turned my face so they wouldn't see me.

"You need a remote detonator," Heather repeated. "Use the remote control unit from a drone. You can get an aerial drone for a couple hundred bucks, online. Cheap. Drive the truck up to the front doors, get out and run like hell for three or four blocks, and then set off the bomb. Fun, hmm?"

I tried to see her, but she was not visible. Strictly audio hallucination. Who the hell *was* Heather? She had become much more than a mere symptom. In comparison, there were the minor voices, with a limited range of subjects to talk about and no real personalities. Sometimes I heard voices from old friends, but these usually did not last long and didn't really have anything to say. Heather, on the other hand, seemed to be into everything I was doing, sometimes as follower and sometimes as leader.

Whatever she had evolved into, she did not have my best

interests in mind.

"Are these destructive thoughts yours…or are they my own ideas?" I asked.

"The elites who made all the money from 9/11 don't care what was real or what was false," she said. "They just want to be rich, and any story it takes to keep the money rolling in, is fair game. What do *you* want?"

This felt like a rebuke. She was right, the situation of mentally ill people in America was horrible, and it was my fault. I had let all these abuses go on too long. Mentally ill people on the streets and in the jails, obviously psychotic and in need of care. You, dear reader, have seen these people walking along the streets and talking to themselves. Sometimes they whisper, sometimes they scream. Sometimes they get in trouble with the cops, or even with you.

On the other hand, President Obama had signed the 21st Century Cures Act into law, and in so doing, he had allocated billions and billions of dollars toward improving the nation's mental health care system.

These facets of the lives of mentally ill people competed in my mind and called up strong emotions. Thirty-six thousand mentally ill people a year committed suicide. I didn't have enough tears to shed for all our losses in this fight, and I couldn't imagine any personal act, such as volunteering at a homeless shelter or a soup kitchen, that would make any real dent in the problem.

Heather offered something else: a straight-up fight, and a life of thunder.

Not everything in my life was negative. I started volunteering at the library again, as a greeter in the small art gallery that was part of the library. I only served for two hours a week, but this activity brought me out around other people and exposed me to lives and viewpoints other than my own.

Heather didn't like it. "These people are probably snitches," she hissed, in some back corner of my mind.

I sat at a desk and greeted people who came into the art gallery and answered questions about the current exhibit. "They're working for the cops, trying to figure out if you're up to something."

Why do you obsess on the cops? I thought.

"You should be thinking about the cops, too. You *should* be planning where to get the materials for a truck bomb. Instead, you see the problem and won't commit to a solution."

A couple of young Asian women came into the art gallery, and I greeted them. Heather shrieked, "GOOKS! FUCKING SLANT-EYED CUNTS!"

My anger at the cops shattered into horror at an ongoing onslaught of slurs.

"DIRTY LITTLE BITCHES!" shouted a minor voice.

"GIVE US SOME PUSSY!" yelped another one.

"FIVE DOLLAR, NO HOLLER!" howled a third voice.

Knock it off! I demanded.

"Put a gun to your head and blow your brains out," said Heather. "That's how you make it stop. Or drive the truck up to police headquarters and stay in the driver's seat while you set off the bomb. Die for your people, damn it."

The Asian women went into the gallery, and Heather and her minor voices shut up.

A couple days after this I took my usual morning walk around my neighborhood, just for sake of exercise. I passed a retirement center, and I walked by some small trees that Parks & Recreation had planted in holes in the sidewalk. A few cars went by, and a small truck pulled up to the curb, but I didn't wait to see its driver get out and unload whatever the truck was carrying for cargo.

Then, very suddenly, I realized I was God. For a few minutes I continued to walk along and reveled in the feeling that I was almighty and omniscient.

A police car cruised past, and its driver seemed to be in something of a hurry. I raised one hand and then brought it down, in an attempt to summon a pillar of fire to smite the cops. When nothing happened, I was sharply disappointed. What was the point of being God if you couldn't smite your enemies?

"Pansy," snapped Heather. "I got that for you, all that power, all that Godhood, and you can't even hang onto it for two minutes."

"It wasn't you," I growled. "It was probably just…"

"What stupid thing are you going to say now?" she goaded.

"It was just…"

"Yes?"

"I don't know," I said.

"When are you going to steal the ingredients for the bomb? When will you steal a truck? Or rent one? *Details!*"

Instead of answering her, I thought of some of the hikes I had taken with friends over the last few months. I pictured California Lilac blossoms, Monkey Flower blooms, and trails turned to mud by winter rains. This was the essence of CBSST techniques, as I employed them: when symptoms start up, think of specific, pleasant things, and try to banish the negative thoughts.

Heather belittled me a few more times, then she disappeared.

Move forward to 7 February, and I woke feeling miserable. I went to the grocery store and bought a bottle of wine and a wedge of cheese and then returned to my room to celebrate having survived eleven years of schizoaffective disorder.

Heather didn't say a thing. I drank the alcohol and read passages out of my first memoir, *Randal, Randal, Burning Bright*. The scenes seemed super-charged, and I was amazed at the bad conditions I had survived and the intensity of the illness that almost got me killed. My goal was not to wallow in pain, misery and loss, but to remember the friends, family, and mental health professionals who had helped me survive such a long period of horror.

Thus, the day was somewhat upbeat and at the same time, very sobering. Yes, I had survived eleven years of hell, but the real point here was that over the years I had tried half a dozen medicines that didn't do much to fight my illness, and I had been under the care of some good psychiatrists. I had told some of my story to family and friends, with an eye to exorcising the illness by talking about it and asking for support when I needed it. My care providers recommended exercise, and so I walked and hiked regularly.

As I drained the last dregs of the bottle, it occurred to me that I did not expect to get better. Not a lot better, not a little better. I could look forward to taking three or four medicines a day, every day, for the rest of my life. Heather and the minor voices would come and go for God knew how long, and they would hassle me with racial slurs, hateful messages, belittling lies, and attempts to get me killed.

That was what I had to look forward to for the rest of my life, be that ten years or twenty. This thought made me feel ill: I had eleven bad years behind me and twenty even worse years in front of me. They would be worse, because I no longer had hope of recovery. Most of my days would include six or eight or ten hours of voices, paranoia, delusions, hallucinations, and generally feeling bad. Every time I opened the paper or scanned news sites on the web I would expect to see that China had pulled out of Tibet, or that the Israelis and the Palestinians had worked out a lasting peace, and I would be cited as the impetus for the olive branch. These delusions that had plagued me for over a decade would continue to follow me, all the way to the grave. Only I, and a few friends who chose to stick it out just to see what happened, would see how the illness progressed.

And, of course, there was always the chance that the symptoms would worsen, and I would sink into utter insanity and spend my final years in an asylum, babbling to the other whack jobs about my mansion in San Francisco, and all my imaginary friends who were famous artists, and my billion dollars that no one had ever seen.

I sent emails to my mentally ill friends and told them what I was up to this wretched day. They answered back that they understood the battles I went through and wished me good luck on taking care of myself and fighting the illness. Kevin told me that he had been bipolar since college, and he suggested I keep trying different medicines until I found one that quieted the voices. Jackie also had been diagnosed bipolar in college, and she said feel free to get in touch any time.

So I got through the day. I tossed the wine bottle in the recycling dumpster outside my building and contemplated my situation.

"Your life will get better," Heather said. She was a buzz in my ear. "You have found your people, and you know who is killing them. Killing *you*. There's a famous quote, you know this one? 'First they came for the Socialists, and I did not speak out—Because I was not a Socialist. Then they came for the Trade Unionists, and I did not speak out— Because I was not a Trade Unionist. Then they came for the Jews, and I did not speak out—Because I was not a Jew. Then they came for me—and there was no one left to speak for me.'"

"I sort of remember that," I muttered.

"The quote comes from a Protestant pastor named Martin Niemöller; he was a critic of Hitler and his policies."

"What happened to him? I imagine Hitler had him killed?"

"Sent him to the concentration camps, yes. He spoke out against Hitler. That wasn't tolerated."

I chewed on that one, and after a bit she said,

"You know who is killing your people and spying on you. What are they planning, once they dummy up enough evidence?"

Fear tore at my guts, and almost right away a fierce anger burned the fear away. "I'm not very political," I mumbled.

Heather ignored this. "You're angry that the cops use your people as cheap sport. Shoot the nut jobs! Beat up thousands of them and throw them in prison! You feel the burn, but you're not ready to get it together and fight back. *When are you going to fight?*"

We went around and around for a while, her pushing me toward violence and me taking the bait and trying to figure out how I'd build the truck bomb.

"Work it out," she commanded. "Nothing more pathetic than a wuss who won't fight for his people."

A day or two went by, and I sat in the café and read a book, when the thought popped into my mind: *I am God.* Immediately I knew it was true; I had only to think about my power, and that power would manifest. The question of course was what to do with it.

Last time I had tried to use Godly power, to smite the cops, nothing happened. The cops continued on their way, I had no fire, and I forgot all about the incident.

This time I thought, *Time for a more positive focus.* I closed my eyes and thought, *Heal all the sick people in the world. Mental illness, physical wounds, all aches and pains and diseases. Do this now.*

Right away I felt really good about the chances for the human race, to get its act together and make something of itself. It was clear I had undersold myself, last time I was God. Petty attacks on authority figures; what a waste of power. Aim for bigger fish!

So I waited for a few minutes, and I noticed no changes in the people around me. If the hundreds of millions of sick and injured people here on earth had mysteriously gotten better, that healing was not obvious to me.

For a second time, I had failed at handling God's power on earth. The feeling of failure piled on the comments Heather had made, about my not being willing to fight the cops, and I wondered what I *was* good at.

Heather piped up, "Suicide bomber. You could do that pretty well. Build the truck bomb, but don't run away from it after you park it outside police headquarters. Stay in the driver's seat and detonate it from there. This will make a man out of you. You'll be an example to mentally ill freedom fighters for a hundred years!"

"Successfully killing a couple hundred cops and living to brag about it will make me a live hero, not a dead memory," I said.

She said nothing, and after a few minutes I realized she had gone away. I could only hope that she would stay away for good, but even as I sent up a little prayer, I knew she would be back.

A few days later I was at the grocery store, picking up food, when I thought of my family walking around Muir Woods, a short drive north of San Francisco. I was maybe eight years old then, my parents in their late twenties, and my brother about five. My dad pointed out the eight-inch long, bright yellow banana slugs that seemed to be all over the place, and there were monarch butterflies here and there, and masses of lady bugs.

I couldn't remember exactly what he said, but I remember feeling like part of something bigger than myself. I was pleased to learn new animals and plants and interesting denizens of nature.

Over the course of my childhood, my family visited dozens if not scores, of parks and preserves. I have fond memories of Yellowstone Park, the Grand Tetons, the San Diego Zoo, White Sands National Monument, the Grand Canyon, and many more.

These memories of course made me miss my father. For the last few years of his cancer he couldn't get around much. I probably should have gone to visit him more frequently, but money was always tight, and it seemed that he would pull out of the death spiral and get a few more years under his belt. That, and I would probably have just spewed delusional nonsense at him and worn him down.

I looked up at the picture of my whole family, taken a few years ago, that hung on my wall over my computer. How my dad was doing in heaven? My mother and my brother and I would meet him there ourselves, one day; hopefully I would get a very long, healthy life, first.

I wished him plenty of hunting trips, to bag those big elk and deer, antelope and wild pig, and maybe even a big horn ram and a moose or two. Good luck, dad, and make friends with the angels.

Over the next few days I continued to work out an outline for the memoir you are currently reading. Work was slow because voices kept plaguing me, and the usual symptoms struck on an almost daily basis. Heather came after me:

"You're not mentally ill; you're lazy. All you do all day is lay around and whine about your symptoms. Whine in emails, whine in letters, whine on the phone, whine on the forums. Everyone needs to support you. What a loser. Killed your own dad with negative thoughts, and now you should kill yourself.

"Oh, by the way; in the past week the cops have killed four more mentally ill people, right here in America. And what did you do to stop them? Where was the counter-attack? When will you stop feeling sorry for yourself and fight back?"

Comments like this made me angry, and it seemed that every day I became a little more aggravated and a little more ready to kill someone. The cops were obviously out of control, and no one could rein them in or make them pay for their murders.

But in the end, it was not the cops who were to blame. Did you blame a rabid German Shepherd for biting people? Did you blame a pit bull for killing other dogs? These animals did what came natural to them, and it was up to people to destroy them. The cops were rabid and violent rogues who had figured out how to game the system so that they never had to pay a price for their crimes.

Holding violent cops to accountability was never going to happen from the inside. Accountability would come from outside, from the community who lost hundreds of people each year.

That meant me.

On the fifteenth of February I went on my normal rounds, but my thoughts were troubled. It was either time to start locating bomb materials, or find some other way to fight.

I sat at my desk and listened to a song from The Cranberries, their song "Zombie," which haunts me every time I hear it. This idea that your head is a battlefield was really close to what I experienced on almost a daily level. I listened to the song about a dozen times, and I started thinking about a story I was working on, where a young Buddhist is offered the chance to become a god--but must go through horrors to achieve apotheosis. I left my apartment and walked a few blocks toward the thrift store, where I wanted to look for a used rain jacket. I got halfway to the store, and it happened.

In that moment psychosis hijacked my mind, and I staggered along the sidewalk, belting out the lyrics to the song. My body filled with energy, tons of energy, and I was seized with the desire to kill *everyone* in a ten-block radius. Incredibly violent fantasies filled my mind, of sending out a psychic shockwave that would drive everyone mad and make them murder each other; I saw a father pick his 4-year-old daughter up by the feet and spin around with her and smash her head into a coffee table, killing her instantly. And the homeless people strangled and beat each other to death. The cops shot all survivors and then turned their weapons on themselves. This was the third time I thought I was God, *and mayhem was good.* Godhood was defined as the ability to destroy maximum numbers of lives. My voices screamed in my head and encouraged me to destroy myself.

It took a while, but I managed to find my way to the thrift store. For a few minutes I went up and down the aisles of clothing, looking for a rain coat, but I could not focus on what I was doing.

"Fuck a rain coat!" shrieked a minor voice. "Buy an umbrella."

"The cops are on to you! FLEE!" shouted another voice.

"Run out into traffic," said a third voice.

I opened my mouth and tried to spit out the voices. Was I mumbling? Shouting? Repeating what the voices had said? I looked around, and it seemed like every person in the store was staring at me. Only a fool would stick around for the cops to show up.

Up the street I went, wanting a slice of pizza, wanting a rain coat, on the lookout for cops, wondering where to find ingredients for truck bombs.

Some of the people on my side of the street looked sketchy. They seemed to be homeless people, some white and some black. If they weren't homeless, what the hell were they doing hanging out on the sidewalk at the middle of the day? So I crossed the street, and here is where things went sour.

I glanced around; I was about to step onto the trolley tracks, and that seemed good. Another man was a few steps behind me. I thought there was something missing, some little habit I was not doing, and I took another step toward the trolley tracks.

There came a blast from the trolley driver's horn, and I glanced that direction. The trolley was no more than twenty feet away from me and approaching fast. Immediately I stepped back and out of harm's way.

In that second, the guy behind me in the crosswalk said, "That's why you want to look where you're going, or they'll kill you."

I said, "No, it's the voices that are trying to kill me."

He stood there and hummed some quiet tune to himself, and we waited for the trolley to go past. I couldn't figure out what had just happened, me stepping on the tracks without looking for the trolley. Was this a suicide attempt? More like 'accidently on purpose.'

No words from Heather in all this, but I was sure she was the mastermind of the day's attempted self-destruction.

Just like that, the episode was over, and I was back in control of myself. I felt worn out and enervated, and I went home and ate a snack and went to sleep.

I dreamed of an incident with the cops in Santa Fe, New Mexico. This was in 2008. I had verbally attacked a woman on a bus, and the bus driver called the cops. I tried to flee, but three cop cars pulled up alongside me. The cops got out, and a young blond cop walked up to me. The other two stayed back a few yards and put their hands on their pistols.

"Bus driver said you are saying weird things," the blond cop said. "Are you stoned, or drunk? Are you hearing voices?"

"Yes, all the time," I said. "Voices making me miserable."

He contemplated this for several seconds. "Do you know about The Life Link?" he asked.

"Never heard of that," I said.

"They treat mental illness, right here in Santa Fe," he said. He gave me an address, and he said, "If you're hearing voices in your head, these people can help you."

Then he and the other officers left, and I sought out the Life

Link and got some help.

Back in 2017 I woke up feeling angry, but not at the cops. The officers in Santa Fe could have shot me, but instead they helped me find my way. Cops as killers, cops as saviors.

"Make up your mind," Heather growled. "It's time to commit to that truck bomb."

And so I did make up my mind. I was done with the cops. I was done with bombs and done with Timothy McVeigh. The *real* asymmetric war was going on in my mind, between my symptoms and my best self. My greatest enemy was not cops but was schizoaffective disorder, and I was confident that if I could beat Heather this time, by refusing to kill people on her command, I could do it again in the future. One little tiny step at a time.

Epilogue

And so it goes. My life is an ongoing struggle against an illness that shows no mercy and takes no prisoners. The down cycles carry me along for months of misery, like a small dog in a flash flood. The up cycles give me hope that one day I will no longer be ill, but let's get real here: I have been schizoaffective for eleven years, and my psychotic symptoms have not improved much.

I found an article online that cited studies of life expectancy for people suffering from severe mental illness. The title of the article was "Life Expectancy in Mental Illness," and in the piece the writer cited a loss of 14 years for people with a severe mental illness.

That is a serious penalty. I will do everything I can to manage my symptoms, but in the end, I expect to be fighting for the rest of my days. It is my heartfelt prayer that I remain stable and do not decline.

I hope that this memoir showed you, dear reader, what it is like to struggle with severe mental illness. My symptoms changed over the eighteen months I covered here. Heather became more powerful, the illness went through cycles of reduced or greater severity, and my delusions became wilder and more grand as time went on.

For all those mentally ill people in prison and on the streets, who God forbid have attempted or even just thought about suicide, I have some idea what you're going through. Find your people, give and accept support, and stay on your medication until you find relief!

ABOUT THE AUTHOR

Randal Doering earned his bachelors degree in English from San Francisco State University and his masters degree in Anthropology from Cal State East Bay. He has written a number of novels and short story collections; you can find out about these at Randal's web site, http://www.rdoering.com.

Randal is the author of two mental illness memoirs: *Randal, Randal, Burning Bright* and *Schizoaffective: Evolution of My Illness*. Both are available on http://www.amazon.com.